AF616423

ADVANCES IN VETERINARY SCIENCE AND COMPARATIVE MEDICINE

VOLUME 31

EXPERIMENTAL AND COMPARATIVE TOXICOLOGY

ADVISORY BOARD

ADVANCES IN VETERINARY SCIENCE AND COMPARATIVE MEDICINE

Edited by

CHARLES E. CORNELIUS
California Primate Research Center
University of California
Davis, California

CHARLES F. SIMPSON
1919–1986

Volume 31

EXPERIMENTAL AND COMPARATIVE TOXICOLOGY

Guest Editor

ANDRÉ G. RICO
Laboratoire de Toxicologie Biochimique et Métabolique (INRA)
Ecole Nationale Vétérinaire
Toulouse, France

1987

ACADEMIC PRESS, INC.
Harcourt Brace Jovanovich, Publishers
Orlando San Diego New York Austin
Boston London Sydney Tokyo Toronto

ACADEMIC PRESS, INC.
Orlando, Florida 32887

United Kingdom Edition published by
ACADEMIC PRESS INC. (LONDON) LTD.
24–28 Oval Road, London NW1 7DX

LIBRARY OF CONGRESS CATALOG CARD NUMBER: 53-7098

ISBN 0–12–039231–3 (alk. paper)

PRINTED IN THE UNITED STATES OF AMERICA

87 88 89 90 9 8 7 6 5 4 3 2 1

CONTENTS

Neurobehavioral Toxicology: An Overview

DAVID L. HOPPER

Immunotoxicology

G. DESCOTES AND G. MAZUÉ

The Endocrine System as the Target in Experimental Toxicology

F. X. R. VAN LEEUWEN, M. A. M. FRANKEN, AND J. G. LOEBER

Uses of γ-Glutamyltransferase in Experimental Toxicology

J. P. BRAUN, G. SIEST, AND A. G. RICO

Predictive Value of Ocular Irritation Tests

PIERRE DUPRAT AND PHILIPPE CONQUET

PREFACE

Experimental toxicology is vital to the assessment of risk caused by the exposure of humans and animals to xenobiotics. Among the latter considered highly significant are certain compounds used by humans, veterinarians, and many others who routinely use pesticides and additives. The objective of this volume is to explore some of these potentially important and crucial areas.

An important problem related to the toxicity of xenobiotics is their potential carcinogenicity. The first three articles are devoted to this topic. If we consider the mechanisms of carcinogenicity, promotion and initiation appear as very key concepts. As Harper and Legator point out in their review, short-term tests should be useful to determine the mode of action of suspected carcinogens. A simplification of methodology, however, is necessary; they propose a "reverse tier" approach as an alternative to extensive *in vitro* assays in which a comprehensive set of genotoxicity tests are performed in individual animals.

The liver is often a target organ for carcinogens. During the experimental production of liver cancer, especially in rodents, several distinct lesions precede the development of malignant tumors. Among such lesions, Williams points out that altered foci are certainly important. He discusses the induction of altered foci, enhancement of altered foci, and inhibition of altered foci as means of detecting carcinogens and identifying neoplasm-promoting agents and anticarcinogens.

During long-term carcinogenicity studies, liver tumors are frequently found in rodents. The problem in such studies is to explain the toxicological significance of such tumors and to extrapolate these results to man. Roe explains and demonstrates that many factors other than test chemicals influence the risk of hepatic neoplasm in laboratory rodents. In light of the data reviewed, calculations of liver tumor risk to humans based on tumor data derived from studies using rodents exposed to very high doses are wholly unreliable from both qualitative and quantitative viewpoints.

Neurobehavioral toxicology is a new and exciting subdiscipline of toxicology. Hopper's contribution defines this new subdiscipline, examines the rationale for studying the effects of toxicants on behavioral processes, discusses the special significance of animal models, and examines test methods and the variables and conditions affecting their use. He also reviews some topics likely to be of future interest and significance to neurobehavioral toxicologists.

The toxicity of xenobiotics to the immune system is also a new area for experimental toxicologists. There are some "classical" models for immunotoxic assessment that explore a variety of different topics such as nonspecific immunity, humoral immunity, cell-mediated immunity, and hypersensitivity reactions. Realistic criteria must soon be defined. Descotes and Mazué provide examples of immune side effects during toxicological studies.

The endocrine system, which is an important integrating system in the mammalian body, can be a target in experimental toxicology. The article by van Leeuwen *et al.* is devoted to this new field. Some practical problems are discussed. Methods of investigation are described and some examples of endocrine toxicological experiments are stressed. For three compounds, bromide, bis(tri-*n*-butyltin) oxide, and β-HCH, immunocytochemical observations and the results of function tests correlate very well and offer a clear picture of the action of endocrine toxic substances.

Enzymology is now a useful tool in pathology for assessing the many potential toxic side effects of xenobiotics. γ-Glutamyltransferase (GGT) is an important enzyme in experimental toxicology. For example, it can be used to explore hepatic biochemical induction mechanisms in species such as ruminants and horses. It is also useful in experimental carcinogenicity testing, especially as a marker for liver tumors. It is also useful in experimental kidney toxicological studies, since urinary GGT is a good test for kidney damage in the proximal tubule.

For many xenobiotics, the determination of their ocular toxicity is needed for their preparation if they are used as human or veterinary drugs or as pesticides. *In vivo* tests for this purpose now exist, especially in rabbits. There has been considerable effort worldwide to develop alternative methods to animal models of ocular irritation, as demonstrated by Duprat and Conquet. It is hoped that new methods will be available soon.

I would like to thank Doctors C. E. Cornelius and C. F. Simpson, who provided me with the opportunity to edit this volume of *Advances in Veterinary Science and Comparative Medicine.* I also appreciate the thoughtful assistance of the staff of Academic Press in compiling this volume and the outstanding contributions of the various authors.

André Rico

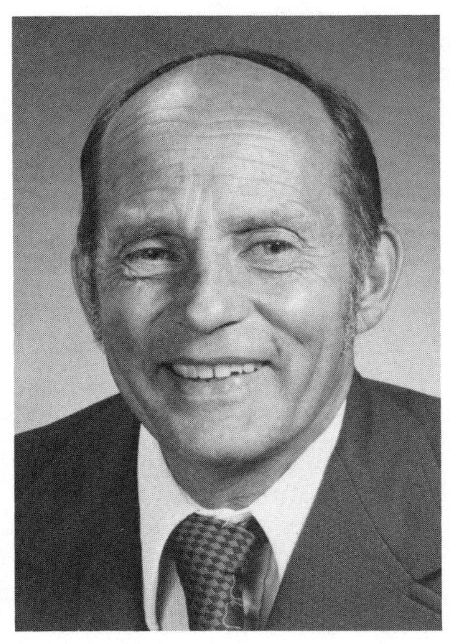

Charles Floyd Simpson
1919–1986

Charles Floyd Simpson
1919–1986

Charles Floyd Simpson was born on January 29, 1919, in East Orange, New Jersey. He received his degree of Doctor of Veterinary Medicine from Cornell University in 1944, a Master of Science in pathology from Ohio State University in 1955 and a Doctor of Philosophy degree, also in pathology, from the University of Minnesota in 1961. Charles joined the Department of Veterinary Science at the University of Florida in 1949 and later transferred to Florida's new College of Veterinary Medicine in 1975, where he served as its first dean for Research. He played a leading role in establishing and developing the College prior to his retirement in 1984.

Dr. Simpson, who coedited *Advances in Veterinary Science and Comparative Medicine* since 1981, gained international recognition for his contributions, as witnessed by over 200 research articles, to both veterinary and human medicine during his 35-year career at the University of Florida. His distinguished studies on hemoprotozoans and cardiovascular-related diseases using the turkey as an animal model resulted in numerous awards: Senior Faculty Research Awards by Gamma Sigma Delta and Sigma Xi in 1969 and 1970, American Veterinary Medicine Association's Research Award in 1970, Fogarty International Fellow in 1977, Florida's Veterinarian of the Year in 1982, outstanding senior faculty researcher at the College of Veterinary Medicine in 1983, and the inaugural Beecham Pharmaceutical Senior Investigator Award in 1984.

Charles was uniquely available and eager to consult with peers on their research projects. His curious but modest approach to helping others on joint projects made him very special and competent in many fields of pathology as witnessed by his publications. As a highly competent electron microscopist, many of his early contributions clarified the pathogenesis of many hemoprotozoan diseases in a wide variety of animal species. His investigations also provided highly significant insights into therapeutic strategies for treating hypertension using hydralazine and propanolol. Dr. Simpson clearly showed that although hydralazine was effective in reducing blood pressure, it could be deleterious to already defective blood vessels. Other studies using turkeys confirmed that the use of propanolol was safe and could at times replace major cardiac surgery in the treatment of aneurysms of the aorta. During the late 1970s, he was first to identify both a herpeslike agent as a killer of a variety of psittacine birds and the encephalomyocarditis virus as the causative agent of fatal heart disease in valuable zoo animals such as the African elephant. His many contributions attest to his selfless dedication to improving human and animal health. We will forever reap the many benefits of his devoted service.

Charles Simpson will long be remembered as a thoughtful and loving father and friend whose strength in human qualities presented a role model to be cherished by us all.

C. E. Cornelius

Tumor Promoters and Genotoxic Chemicals in Short-Term Testing for Carcinogenicity

BARBARA L. HARPER AND MARVIN S. LEGATOR

Division of Environmental Toxicology, Department of Preventive Medicine and Community Health, University of Texas Medical Branch, Galveston, Texas 77550

I. Introduction

The ultimate goal of toxicity testing, including genetic toxicology and carcinogenicity evaluation, is to predict and therefore prevent adverse human health effects. Hopefully, this can be accomplished in animals before significant exposure levels in humans have occurred. Inherent problems with human epidemiology make it difficult to detect any but the most potent, site-specific, and/or widespread carcinogens. Ethical and practical considerations mandate the use of multiple short-term animal tests for the detection and characterization of carcinogens. Extrapolation from animals to humans presents some quantitative difficulties but not qualitative ones. Some species are more sensitive to certain kinds of carcinogens due to metabolic differences, and some are more sensitive at one target site than another, but our existing data base would indicate that animal carcinogens are all potential human carcinogens.

A major difficulty in assessing risks and setting exposure limits is our lack of understanding of carcinogenic mechanisms. This leads us, correctly, to require large safety factors when extrapolating from animals to humans. Recently, there has been a trend for regulatory agencies to assume that, at comparable dose levels and apparent potency, some carcinogens are safer than others (reviewed by Perera, 1984; Harper and Morris, 1984; Hooper, 1984). This problem, largely a matter of semantics, arose in part because short-term mutagenicity tests that are used to predict carcinogenic potential were developed and validated using the carcinogens which had been identified at that time, namely potent alkylating agents. Since then, a number of bacterial false-negatives, or animal carcinogens that are not detected in bacterial mutagenicity systems, have been identified. Bacterial validation experiments may be designed to detect 100% or 0% of a set of carefully selected chemicals, if there is unequal distribution between chemical classes. On the whole, the *Salmonella*/microsome assay detects approximately 70–75% of animal carcinogens (Rinkus and Legator, 1980; Zeiger and Tennant, 1985). Some of these bacterial nonmutagens are, in reality, weak mutagens and/or weak carcinogens, and have been designated "epigenetic" carcinogens (Williams, 1983a,b; Weisburger and Williams, 1983). with the assumption that "epigenetic" carcinogenesis has a threshold, and therefore that epigenetic carcinogens are safer at low levels than "genotoxic" carcinogens.

There are a number of reasons why carcinogens are not detected as bacterial mutagens. Some of these reasons are metabolic in nature: complex *in vivo* metabolism which is not duplicated by liver homogenates, *in vivo–in vitro* differences such as interactions between organs or tissues, and organ-specific metabolism or sensitivities (Rinkus and Legator, 1980; Ward *et al.,* 1981). Noncovalent binding to DNA may also cause damage that may or may not be detected in bacteria, such as that caused by intercalating agents or high-dose-level ionic binding (Ashby, 1983a). Other agents damage DNA indirectly by generating radicals or hydrogen peroxide, and newer definitions of "epigenetic" carcinogens include this damage as genotoxic rather than epigenetic, even when there is no covalent binding to DNA. Some agents bind preferentially to proteins such as nuclear protein or tubulin, and cause aneuploidy or mitotic interference rather than point mutations. Other agents, such as those causing metabolic deficiencies, may enhance the rate of spontaneous mutations, while others, such as direct inhibitors of repair or agents which affect the fidelity of repair, increase the likelihood of nonrepair or misrepair. The use of the term epigenetic in most cases merely signifies that we do not know or understand the mechanism by which genetic alterations are induced. The failure of a chemical to induce mutation *in vitro* should not be used as a factor in risk assessment when *in vivo* studies are positive; in fact, there is a distinct possibility that unique activity *in vivo* is highly significant.

Some investigators advocate a battery of only *in vitro* tests in order to reduce the need of long-term bioassays, but it is obvious that a minimum battery of *in vivo* tests is necessary to detect carcinogens arising wholly or partially through the above-mentioned mechanisms.

Fortunately, carcinogenicity bioassays of some of these "epigenetic" chemicals did not wait for positive evidence of mutagenicity in *in vitro* tests.

Because of the variety of mechanisms involved in inducing DNA damage, it is probably improper to try to make a distinction between direct and indirect genotoxicity. Other problems with defining epigenetic carcinogens have been discussed before (Harper and Morris, 1984; Perera, 1984; Ashby, 1983a) and can be dealt with by defining carcinogens as agents which always ultimately affect the structure, integrity, or expression of DNA (Ashby, 1983a), regardless of whether direct or indirect mechanisms are involved. In other words, an "epigenetic" carcinogen of a given potency should not be assumed to be safer than a "genotoxic" carcinogen of the same potency (Perera, 1984).

For the category of chemicals usually listed as epigenetic carcinogens, we are distinguishing complete carcinogens from pure promoters or agents with much stronger promoting than initiating activity (ICPEMC, 1984). Many of these so-called epigenetic carcinogens are carcinogenic only at prolonged high doses, and it is difficult to distinguish between weak but complete carcinogens, and pure promoters such as phenol and phenobarbital. Since some promoters also have weak genotoxicity, it is hard to say whether such promoters are really complete carcinogens with a low initiating potential, or whether they are promoting preexisting lesions. Some of these "epigenetic" carcinogens are detected only at cytotoxic doses, and therefore it is inferred that cytotoxicity is a major mechanism of their carcinogenicity. However, while cytotoxicity may be required for their actions, it is not sufficient for carcinogenicity, as seen by the number of cytotoxic agents which neither initiate nor promote cancer. The real question is whether "safe" levels of these carcinogens exist.

Some of the agents that operate through indirect mechanisms may have thresholds, particularly those that require long-term, high-dose exposure at cytotoxic levels to cause tumors, usually detected as mouse liver cancer. These thresholds, however, may be theoretical, apparent, or real (Ehling *et al.*, 1983; Sobels, 1984). Theoretical thresholds may exist for repair of DNA lesions, but this repair is sometimes cited as if it is perfect (Reitz and Watanabe, 1983). In reality, a substantial body of evidence exists that indicates that regulation of error-free repair is a function of the length of the cell cycle (reviewed by Trosko and Chang, 1981). We must also assume constant human exposure to inhibitors of repair, such as caffeine. In addition, repair is saturable, and we cannot assume that there is no concomitant subthreshold damage from exposure to low levels of other chemicals. This is especially true in reference to individual chemicals that are being considered relatively safe because they may cause only lesions that are likely to be repaired.

Another problem with thresholds is that they are measured epidemiologically as the "dose limit over which no significant biological effect *can be recognized* within the lifetime of the species" (Higginson, 1983, emphasis added). This author does not say that a threshold is the level below which an effect does not occur. Particularly in human epidemiology, an *apparent* threshold may not be the same as a *true* threshold, because of the difficulties in proving a negative. It should be assumed that, at a minimum, effects of genotoxic carcinogens should be summated, so that any exposure, no matter how small, carries a potential risk. As yet, there is no standardized way of taking into account genetic variability, presence of modulating factors, and so on, for the purposes of risk assessment (Ehling *et al.*, 1983).

II. Complete and "Incomplete" Carcinogens

A. Promoters and Antipromoters

Several models of carcinogenicity have been proposed, both for understanding mechanisms and designing therapy, and for regulatory purposes. For example, multistage models of initiation–promotion or initiation–promotion–selection have been demonstrated experimentally and are useful in examining specific factors which may modify each step. Multihit mutational models have been used in determining biologically effective doses necessary to cause mutation or tumor formation, and in reverse to determine allowable exposure levels. Of course, different agents do not all cause cancer in the same way, and data do not fit into a single integrative theory. We assume that promotion occurs in humans as well as in animals, and that most human cancer is multifactorial and/or multichemical in causation (Yamasaki, 1984; Ramel, 1984). Smoking, for example, is synergistic with other exposures, although it is impossible to distinguish the effects of the promoters, initiators, and cocarcinogens which are all present in cigarette smoke. Similarly, other risk factors are being identified for different types of cancer which may be partly promotional in nature, such as dietary fat, vitamin deficiency, excess bile salts, hormonal factors, and so on. Removal of some of these risk factors, such as smoking cessation, diminishes the risk, satisfying part of the definition of promotion, namely reversibility.

Early work with mouse skin carcinogens indicated that an irreversible event was necessary as a first step, defined as initiation or mutation. Expression of this genetic event can then proceed through two stages of promotion, portions of which are partially reversible if the promoting agent is removed before the promoted state becomes fixed. This process has been identified in many organs and appears to be a general phenomenon (Slaga and DiGiovani, 1984; many others). In the first stage of promotion, a single application of a stage I promoter such as TPA, H_2O_2, calcium ionophore A23187, or wounding, is sufficient. Specific inhibitors for stage I include antiinflammatory agents and protease inhibitors, which prevent some of the hyperplasia and polyamine synthesis. This really explains little about the mechanisms of tumor formation, since hyperplastic agents are not necessarily promoters (Slaga, 1983; Slaga and Digiovanni, 1984; Slaga and Fischer, 1985; Trosko and Chang, 1981; Pitot and Sirica, 1980). Stage II of promotion appears to be initially reversible, then becomes irreversible upon sufficient application of a stage II promoter. Specific biochemical events have been identified for stage II, and specific inhibitors are known, but again, none of these are specific to tumor formation.

The nonspecificity of promoters and antipromoters is exemplified by several agents which may act in either role, depending on the dose and sequence of application with respect to the initiator, such as phenobarbital, retinoids, BHA, and many of the chlorinated hydrocarbon mouse liver tumor promoters (or complete carcinogens), such as DDT, TCDD, and PCBs (Slaga and Digiovanni, 1984). Similarly, antipromoters may inhibit some tumors but not others, which may be a function of the tissue specificity of the carcinogen, the promoter, and the antipromoter. Furthermore, antipromoters do not block carcinogenesis by a complete carcinogen at a specific stage of antipromotion, indicating that mechanisms exist to bypass requirements for specific promotional steps. Complete carcinogenesis in this case implies that the entire process has already been programmed into the DNA ("self-promotion," Ashby, 1983a) and that the process might be delayed by antipromoters but not reversed. A final question concerns the difference between a single initiating but subcarcinogenic dose of a complete carcinogen, which requires the application of a promoter or more carcinogen for the initial neoplastic mutation to be expressed, and a single larger dose of the same chemical which is completely carcinogenic without the need for promoters. This phenomenon has been demonstrated for X rays (Larsson, 1984) and for many chemicals.

Free Radicals and Promotion

The role of free radicals in both initiation and promotion has been the topic of much discussion. There is no doubt that radicals, and especially reactive oxygen metabolites, can result in chromosome aberrations, mutagenesis, and modulation of gene expression, and that promoters often increase radical production (Emerit and Cerutti, 1982; Cerutti *et al.*, 1983a,b, 1985; Parke and Ioannides, 1984; Popper, 1984). Mechanisms by which certain promoters increase radical production include induction of membrane oxidases, peroxisomes, and electron transport in mitochondria and endoplasmic reticulum (Kensler and Trush, 1984; Ashby, 1983a; Reddy *et al.*, 1983). The specific targets involved in initiation or promotion remain undefined, except in broad terms. Some active oxygen forms are complete carcinogens, and some initiate only weakly if at all (Cerutti, 1985). Different oxygen forms are also specific for different stages of promotion, because specific radical scavengers may inhibit only one stage of promotion or another, and because low or subcarcinogenic–submutagenic doses of radical-generating agents, such as X rays, may not substitute for specific promoters (Schwarz *et al.*, 1984). Finally, although promotion by radicals may be involved with sister chromatid exchange (SCE) generation and translocation (Ashby, 1983a), the question still remains how radicals, with half-lives of less than a millisecond, promote as well as initiate (Willson, 1982).

B. Membrane-Mediated Effects and Oncogenes

Many phenomena associated with transformation are interrelated through membrane-mediated effects, including involvement of receptors and protein kinase C, lipid peroxidation, metabolic cooperation, dietary fat and associated membrane lipid composition, and enzyme induction. Many of these effects may be promotional in nature, but the agents involved may also have some genotoxicity via radical production or altered bioactivation of other carcinogens. There is also some overlap with enhanced oncogene expression, since some of the receptor-mediated events caused by carcinogens or promoters involve oncogene products (discussed below). However, none of these events is specific to promotion or transformation, so while they may be necessary events in certain instances, they are not sufficient for the production of cancer. As an example, some strains of mice (Sencar) are more sensitive to carcinogens, and have higher background rates of tumors. However, treatment with an initiating agent is still required for tumor production, and treatment with 12-*O*-tetradecanoyl-phorbol-13-acetate (TPA) does not cause increased conversion of papillomas to carcinomas over spontaneous conversion rates, so even this sensitive strain does not appear to have more initiated cells or to be unusually promotable (Yuspa, 1983).

A role of metabolic cooperation during promotion has been suggested by the observations that it is inhibited by many promoters, including TPA (Enomoto *et al.*, 1981; Walder and Lutzelschwab, 1984) and some of the liver carcinogens/promoters discussed below such as DDT, lindane, and chlordane (Tshushimoto *et al.*, 1983), as well as unsaturated dietary fatty acids (Aylsworth *et al.*, 1984; Trosko *et al.*, 1982). It is not clear how cooperation relates to other membrane-mediated effects, especially peptide receptors and associated phospholipid metabolism, but research is in progress.

Membrane phospholipids, and phosphoinositides in particular, act as signal transmitters for certain hormones, growth factors, and neurotransmitters. There is evidence connecting this sytem to uncontrolled growth and other aberrant effects of oncogenes (Marx, 1985; Nishizuka, 1984a,b; Kensler and Trush, 1984; Blumberg *et al.*, 1984; Josephs *et al.*, 1984; Duesberg, 1985). Receptor binding causes generation of inositol triphosphate and diacylglycerol; this step is possibly mediated by an enzymatic product of the *ras* oncogene. Diacylglycerol in turn activates protein kinase C, as well as inhibiting gap junctional communication (Gainer and Murray, 1985). Oleic or linoleic acids increase the pool of diacylglycerol (Homa *et al.*, 1983), and the arachidonate cascade may also be involved in the activation of protein kinase C (McPhail *et al.*, 1984; Slaga and Fischer, 1985, and references therein). Eventually, a signal to divide is transmitted to the nucleus, possibly by an isomer of inositol triphosphate which has a sufficient half-life to reach the nucleus (reviewed by Marx, 1985). Oncogenes are involved at several points in the process (reviewed by Kris *et al.*, 1985). One of the polypeptide chains of PDGF is encoded by the *sis* oncogene and may represent an oncogene family expressed as the mediators. Receptors for EGF, PDGF, IGF-1, and insulin are glycoproteins and members of the *src* family of oncogenes. These receptors, when bound with the mediator, display tyrosine kinase activity, and self-phosphorylate as well as phosphorylating other proteins. Diacylglycerol generation, possibly involving the *ras* family products as "coupling factors" in hormone receptor systems, activates protein kinase C, which phosphorylates at Ser and Thr residues. Products of the *myc, myb,* and *fos* oncogenes are nuclear proteins apparently involved in differentiation and cell cycle progression.

Expression of the various oncogene products may be influenced by many things, resulting in up-regulation or down-regulation. Self-phosphorylation of the receptors, for example, results in down-regulation by decreasing the affinity of the receptor for the ligand. Promoters activating protein kinase C would also cause down-regulation due to increased receptor phosphorylation, but many nonpromoters and cytochrome *P*-450 inducers also cause down-regulation of EGF receptors (Karenlampis *et al.,* 1983) as well as inducing choline kinase and causing an increase in the choline phosphate pool (Ishidate *et al.,* 1982).

Oncogene mutations, insertions, internal rearrangements, and gene translocations have been identified as contributing to particular states of neoplastic sensitivity or to *in vitro* transformation (reviewed by Varmus, 1984). Chemically transformed fibroblast cell lines may express high levels of the proto-*myc* product without translocation or internal rearrangement, while some Burkitt's lymphoma cell lines have mutated and translocated but not internally rearranged *myc* genes. This mutation sometimes is and sometimes is not involved in *myc* activation (Duesberg, 1985). Alkylating agents activate a *ras* oncogene in fetal guinea pig cells associated with the acquisition of tumorigenicity (Sukumar *et al.,* 1984). In another system, transforming activity was due to one point mutation in the *ras* gene acquired during passage of host PA1 teratocarcinoma cells. The transformed cells also carried a translocation and a non-*ras* transforming gene, but their presence preceded the *ras* mutation, focus formation, and transforming ability (Tainsky *et al.,* 1984). Colburn *et al.* (1982, 1984) also postulated the presence of additional transforming genes in JB6 cells, one of which appeared to be required for increased sensitivity to promotion, and one for maintenance of promotion. Her colleagues also tentatively identified a protein essential for transformation as a heat stress protein (Gindhart *et al.,* 1984).

Altered expression rather than an altered gene product also occurs in some instances of transformation. As suggested by Ashby (1983b), translocation, measured by SCE, rather than mutation may be the stimulus to altered expression in these cases. For example, a Burkitt's lymphoma cell line has been isolated which carries a translocation upstream of the *myc* gene, resulting in altered expression (Wiman *et al.,* 1984). Constitutive fragile sites, whose fragility is increased by agents such as caffeine, may be involved in human cancer (Yunis and Soreng, 1984). While such translocations may enhance tumorigenicity, they are not always necessary, as exemplified by other Burkitt's lines which do not have actively expressed or translocated *myc* genes (Duesberg, 1985).

The controversy concerning mouse liver tumor promotion has included the suggestion that these hepatocytes are either already initiated, prone to initiation upon exposure, or easily promoted possibly due to ease of translocation or to easily activated oncogenes. The implication is that human hepatocytes are not easily transformed, and therefore mouse liver-only carcinogens should be considered safer for humans than mouse multiorgan carcinogens (Fox and Watanabe, 1985). As pointed out by Yunis and Soreng (1984) and Murphree and Benedict (1984), however, easily activated oncogenes or constitutively fragile sites do exist in the human genome, and certain genetic conditions (retinoblastoma, for example) may be analogous to the mouse liver system with respect to sensitivity to transformation.

C. Alkylation and Other Genotoxic versus Indirect Effects

The distinction between direct and indirect genetic damage is further blurred by examples of alkylation of proteins involved in DNA conformation, such as topoisomerases, and high-dose ionic binding to DNA as discussed by Ashby (1983b). Agents known to alkylate other proteins such as hemoglobin include a number of the "epigenetic" carcinogens in question, including chloroform, carbon tetrachloride, 1,2-dichloroethane, and benzene (Calleman, 1984). How much of this binding is paralleled by specific and critical DNA binding is not clear, however. For example, benzene, a moderate clastogen, or its metabolites, binds to DNA at low levels, but since benzene's metabolites are only weakly clastogenic at best, much of this binding must be irrelevant to chromosome damage. Its metabolites include phenol, a promoter, and DNA binding of this metabolite may be related to promotion more than to initiation. Hydroquinone, another benzene metabolite, is a weakly clastogenic metabolite of phenol, and it binds to sulfhydryl groups, most notably in tubulin, causing spindle damage and sequelae. Other agents also cause aneuploidy but not mitotic crossing over or point mutations in yeast by causing spindle fiber microtubule malfunction (Zimmerman *et al.,* 1985). Intercalating agents are well known to cause structural DNA damage without covalently binding. Other agents such as epipodophyllotoxins do not even intercalate but still cause single and double strand breaks, possibly involving DNA topoisomerase II (Tewey *et al.,* 1984), while other agents such as UV radiation and psoralens cause structural distortion which may also interfere with expression or mitosis.

The specificity of adducts, both large and small, and their relevance to transformation, has been the subject of numerous studies. In particular, the persistence of O^6-Me-guanine or O^6-Et-guanine correlates well with carcinogenic potency of ethylating and methylating agents (Lawley, 1979; Bartsch *et al.*, 1983; Hemminki, 1983), because these adducts cause the most mispairing (Swenson, 1983). The N^7-guanine position is the most nucleophilic site, and is preferentially alkylated by larger agents, while polyaromatic hydrocarbons form N^2-guanine adducts, and aromatic amines form C^8-guanine adducts (Swenson, 1983; Hemminki, 1983). Even the presence of specific adducts, however, is not sufficient for transformation. On the one hand, O^6-Et-guanine adducts formed by ethylnitrosourea (ENU) accumulate in the rat brain, the primary organ at risk for tumors in the rat, because they are less easily repaired than the same adducts that occur in the liver. The mouse brain has just as little repair as the rat brain, however, but is not as susceptible to ENU or practically any other chemical. Conversely, higher levels of the specific repair enzyme, O^6-methyl transferase, exist in the liver, an organ at greater risk (Kliehues *et al.*, 1983). The level of methylation appears to be correlated with gene expression of some genes, but while alkylation is associated with hypermethylation, some genes are active only when undermethylated, while for others it makes no difference (Ashby, 1983a); thus methyl adducts may only be effective in altering expression in a subset of genes, while other genes may be affected only by point mutations requiring cell division for fixation.

III. Acute and Chronic Toxicity

A. Differences in Target Tissues

Many of the chemicals that have been designated as epigenetic are chlorinated hydrocarbons which cause direct neurotoxicity after acute exposure, and liver tumors, especially in mice, after chronic exposures at high doses. The liver tumors may be the result of complete carcinogenesis or promotion of preexisting initiated cells, but at present there is no real mechanism for distinguishing between the two. Although chronic toxicity appears to be involved with some liver neoplasias, it is clearly not the overriding mechanism of tumor induction, or the tumors would develop in the primary target tissue showing acute toxic effects of these agents: the brain or central nervous system (CNS). Similarly, many hepatotoxins are not liver carcinogens or promoters, and the most potent hepatotoxins are not the most potent hepatocarcinogens. Several suggestions may be made to explain this discrepancy:

1. Based on background rates of mouse liver tumors compared to CNS neoplasms, the probability of detecting a rare event such as cancer is much higher in the liver than in the CNS, which has a very low spontaneous incidence.

2. The mouse brain may be intrinsically resistant to initiation or promotion, as very few potent carcinogens cause mouse brain tumors.

3. Comparison of chlorinated and nonchlorinated hydrocarbons may indicate a structure–activity relationship with respect to target tissues and neoplasia versus toxicity.

Spontaneous rates of liver tumors in male BCF mice ranges from 7 to 58%, with a 32% average over different laboratories and different experiments, and female mice average 6.2% (Tarone *et al.*, 1981; Hamm, 1984). Spontaneous rates of mouse brain cancer were 0.07% (2/2543) in male BCF mice, and 0.06% (2/2522) in female mice (Ward *et al.*, 1979). In a review of many experiments using a total of over 77,000 mice of different strains, the brain tumor incidence was 0.07% in control mice and 0.05% in treated mice, and many of these tumors were lipomas, which are not considered true neoplasms by some investigators (Morgan *et al.*, 1984). Mouse brain tumors have been induced by very few chemicals, such as 1,3-butadiene (Huff *et al.*, 1985) and ENU (Vesselinovitch *et al.*, 1977; Wechsler *et al.*, 1979). The reviews of the National Cancer Institute (NCI) bioassays (Griesemer and Cueto, 1980; Haseman *et al.*, 1984) list the sites of tumor formation, and many carcinogens caused tumors in mouse liver, while only a very few of even the most potent multiorgan carcinogens caused brain tumors. The statistical power of bioassays to detect a doubling over a background incidence of 1 per 1000, when 50 animals per group are at risk, is nil. With a sample size of 50 animals per group, a doubling can only be measured in organs with a reasonable (15%) background incidence. This limits detection in organs with lower background incidences, and any tumor arising in these tissues is cause for concern even though statistics cannot be applied. The NCI Bioassay Reports do report such rare tumors as potentially important, but regulatory agencies, of course, need actual numbers to determine relative risk. Thus the probability of detecting a statistically significant increase over these background rates is much higher for liver than any other site; this might actually be an advantage to both mechanistic and screening studies (Stevens and Peraino, 1983). A different argument can be made concerning whether to maximize the probability of detection of potential carcinogens by using the most sensitive strains and tissues, or to approximate an average sensitivity which might be more realistic to human exposures (Ashby, 1982; deSerres and Ashby, 1981).

Although the cancer rates differ greatly between the liver and brain in mice, there are as many or more CNS toxins as liver toxins. Many of the hepatotoxins are chlorinated hydrocarbons, while many of the CNS depressants are solvents (Dukes, 1980; Hughes, 1978; Daugaard, 1978). Some toxicity is due to direct effects on membranes or to direct alkylation of proteins or DNA, while other toxicity requires bioactivation of the chemical and/or participation of generated radicals. Specific chemicals causing liver cancer are frequently enzyme inducers, and are lipophilic, immunosuppressive, and neurotoxic; thus they cause general membrane and multitissue toxicity, but are detected as carcinogens only in the liver. Some may be both carcinogens and anticarcinogens (such as DDT; Kitagawa *et al.,* 1984b), depending on the regimen used.

One interesting pair of chemicals is benzene and chlorobenzene–bromobenzene. The acute effect of benzene is neurotoxicity, while chronic effects include bone marrow and immune suppression and various cancers in mice (NTP report No. 289) and leukemia in humans. It is clastogenic in single doses at 3–10 *M,* or 0.1–0.5 *M* in subacute or chronic exposures. The liver, while it metabolizes benzene, does not appear to be a target tissue. On the other hand, chlorobenzene is an irritant and CNS depressant, and causes liver, kidney, and blood damage. Bromobenzene is a classic hepatotoxin, causing centrilobular necrosis, as well as nervous and immune suppression and lung and kidney damage. Bromobenzene and chlorobenzene, while causing liver toxicity, are not markedly carcinogenic in this or any other organ, while benzene, which is less toxic, causes multiorgan carcinogenicity. This may be partly because it is possible to test less toxic chemicals at higher prolonged doses than more toxic chemicals. Although fewer tumors occurred in the livers of benzene-treated mice than in those treated with many other chemicals, benzene actually caused tumors in more sites than any of the chemicals reviewed by Haseman *et al.* (1984). It is widely assumed that epoxide intermediates of benzene and halogenated benzenes are the toxic metabolites, at least with respect to clastogenicity, but other toxicity involving direct membrane effects may also involve cell division, saturated detoxification and repair, and so on. For example, bromobenzene causes a direct increase of phospholipase C activity in membranes, mediating a Ca^{2+}-dependent increase in diacylglycerol concentration, without any metabolism being required, while benzene has no such effect (Lamb and Schwertz, 1982).

Organochlorine pesticides as a class are frequently used as examples of mouse liver epigenetic carcinogens. They are designed to be neurotoxic, but they also have many other effects. Most (lindane, DDT, many others) are phenobarbital-type liver enzyme inducers, and cause associated morphological changes after chronic exposure (Chambers and Yarbrough, 1982), as well as causing degeneration in many tissues (Hayes, 1982; Sittig, 1981; Toxicology Data Base). These chemicals are widely distributed in the body, including the brain (which is obvious from their CNS depressant activity) and the liver (Eichler *et al.*, 1983; Toxicology Data Base). Tumors are limited to the liver, however, even though other organs have higher levels of the chemicals and more associated cytotoxicity (IARC, 1979; Harper *et al.*, 1983), so there may be some intrinsically increased promotability in the mouse liver that other tissues do not share. This may be related in part to the increased numbers of TPA receptors found in rat brain relative to the liver (reviewed in Weinstein, 1981) or increased numbers of growth factor receptors in mouse brain, as well as to a lower rate of metabolic activation or repair, although neither explanation is sufficient by itself.

B. Liver Tumor Promotion

A good deal of controversy still exists concerning whether mouse liver tumors represent complete carcinogenesis or pure promotion, and which lesions represent neoplasia or preneoplasia. Many or most investigators now consider altered enzyme foci to be preneoplastic in that some foci progress even though many regress (Farber, 1980). The foci which do progress either spontaneously or after treatment with the carcinogen–promoter, however, must by definition have been initiated at some point, whether spontaneously or chemically. On the other hand, single treatments of complete carcinogens must cause enough genetic changes to result eventually in "self-promotion" (Ashby, 1983a). Mouse liver carcinogens have many cellular effects, and even pure promoters such as phenobarbital cause a variety of effects, such as enzyme induction, nonspecific mitogenesis (Peraino *et al.*, 1983; Yuyan and Zhen, 1985), changes in ploidy and atypical nuclear figures, and generation of hydrogen peroxide and superoxygen anions (Kunz *et al.*, 1983). Ploidy changes could change heterozygous mutations into homozygous ones (Kunz *et al.*, 1983), or remove oncogene transsuppressors. Some models suggest that mitogenic stimulation increases the probability of a second mutation involved in promotability, or that both types of mutations occur with sufficient doses of complete carcinogens but not with subcarcinogenic doses. Alternately, promotion could involve SCEs, representing altered expression rather than altered base sequences, which would have a theoretical threshold (Ashby, 1983a).

Promotion of preexisting genetic lesions or preneoplastic foci must exist in parallel to multiple-mutation mechanisms. Altered enzyme foci increase with age at a high enough incidence in putatively unexposed rats to suggest that there must be a genetically programmed mechanism involved in focus generation (Popp *et al.,* 1985; Schulte-Herman *et al.,* 1983b). Many mouse liver carcinogens accelerate the enlargement of preexisting microfoci as well as increasing detectable focus numbers (Schulte-Herman *et al.,* 1983a), supporting the argument that initiated foci arise spontaneously. On the other hand, a morphological examination of potential preneoplastic lesions suggests that focal basophilic hyperplasia is related to spontaneous liver carcinomas (which are mostly basophilic), and that true promotion therefore should increase the incidence only of basophilic carcinomas. Mouse liver carcinogens, however, produce basophilic and eosinophilic tumors in approximately equal ratios, suggesting that more than just promotional mechanisms are involved in mouse liver carcinogenesis (Ward, 1984).

Hepatotoxicity and Hepatocarcinogenicity

Types of hepatotoxicity are based on the cells involved and the kind of damage produced, and no particular type of toxicity, either acute or chronic, is consistently related to carcinogenicity (Zimmerman, 1980, 1982; Newberne, 1982; Mitchell *et al.,* 1984; Leonard *et al.,* 1983). While some cytotoxicity is caused directly, not requiring metabolism of the chemical, most is caused by reactive metabolites and active radicals produced during metabolism of the chemical. Superoxide and hydroxyl radicals cause lipid peroxidation and associated membrane effects, and radical intermediates of halogenated hydrocarbons and other chemicals cause similar effects. The question still remains why the mouse liver is uniquely susceptible to halogenated hydrocarbons even though many or most tissues are exposed and affected during distribution and metabolism of these chemicals. One possibility is reductive dechlorination, which can occur in the normal liver (Baker *et al.,* 1985; Tsushimoto *et al.,* 1983; Frank *et al.,* 1982; Reynolds and Moslen, 1980; Tomasi *et al.,* 1984).

IV. New Testing Strategies

The consensus of the many reports concerning batteries of short-term genotoxicity tests for predicting carcinogenicity is that *in vitro* tests by themselves are not sufficient (Food Safety Council, 1980; National Toxicology Program, 1984; other programs). It has been suggested that fewer expensive and time-consuming rodent lifetime bioassays could be performed by relying on *in vitro* tests for prediction (Weisburger and Williams, 1981; Weisburger and Wynder, 1984).

Considering the number of *in vitro*-negative animal carcinogens, however, a more realistic approach is to rely on *in vivo* tests as a surrogate (Ashby, 1983a). No matter what the testing mix or how extensive the *in vitro* assays are, they will not satisfy the necessary requirements for testing. These requirements are (1) the need to evaluate *in vivo* complex metabolic steps and (2) organ and tissue specificity. We propose that a "reverse-tier" approach be employed as an alternate to extensive *in vitro* screening, in which a comprehensive set of genotoxicity tests are performed in individual animals. A number of genotoxicity tests in somatic and reproductive cells can be combined into a single protocol so that effects in each target tissue can be compared within the same animal. We are currently combining bone marrow metaphase and micronucleus analysis, spleen lymphocyte cytogenetics, point mutation and labeling index analysis, spermatocyte cytogenetic analysis, pulmonary alveolar macrophage cytogenetic analysis, peripheral erythrocyte micronucleus analysis, liver enzyme analysis, and liver and lung histopathology. Comparative results after low-dose exposures to a gas mixture will be reported elsewhere. This combined testing protocol approach is efficient and economic, and examines several potential target tissues simultaneously.

This battery may be used for any chemical with wide or chronic human exposure, and might be used in conjunction with a conventional *Salmonella*/microsome assay, as proposed by Ashby (1982, 1983b). *In vitro* testing would be used to generate additional information, particularly concerning mechanisms of genotoxicity. An in-depth analysis of the mutagenic, carcinogenic potential is generated in which several (8–10) separate assays are performed in individual animals, including the induction of genetic damage in both somatic and germinal cells. The results of a first-level animal study are prerequisite to undertaking further studies of metabolism and mechanism of action. The time has come to reverse our thinking; that is, instead of going from simple (*in vitro*) to complex testing (*in vivo*), we must go from complex to simple.

V. Conclusions

Based on the present discussion, we would draw the same conclusion that other investigators and working groups have drawn: that insufficient data exist to support attempts to predict carcinogenic risk based on mechanisms of carcinogenicity. If a chemical is carcinogenic, regulation should be based on "categories of concern," which in turn are derived from mutagenic, clastogenic, carcinogenic, or teratogenic potency *in vivo*. An apparently complete carcinogen in one system should be regarded as a potential complete carcinogen in other systems. Assumptions of thresholds, reversibility, and, therefore, relative safety should not be made for known carcinogens, regardless of the site of tumor formation, although such assumptions are reasonable for clearly identified pure promoters. Assurance of pure promoting without initiating ability has been realized for a few chemicals and only after extensive *in vivo* and *in vitro* work. Without well-validated screening tests for promotion, there is at present no simple way of distinguishing between promoters and complete carcinogens. For human safety, then, carcinogens are assumed to be complete carcinogens until proven otherwise. The contributions of synergism, protection, multiple exposures, and individual sensitivities cannot be quantitated, and will often lead to an underestimation of risk.

References

Ashby, J. (1982). *In* "Mutagenicity: New Horizons in Genetic Toxicology" (John A. Heddle, ed.), pp. 1–31. Academic Press, New York.

Ashby, J. (1983a). *In* "Current Problems in Drug Toxicology" (G. Zbinden and J. Y. Detaille, eds.), pp. 200–223. Libbey, London.

Ashby, J. (1983b). *Mutat. Res.* **115,** 177–213.

Aylsworth, C. *et al.* (1984). *J. Natl. Cancer Inst.* **72,** 637–645.

Baker, M. T. *et al.* (1985). *Arch. Biochem. Biophys.* **236,** 506–514.

Bartsch, H. *et al.* (1983). *Mutat. Res.* **110,** 181–219.

Blumberg, P. M. *et al.* (1984). *Biochem. Pharmacol.* **33,** 933–940.

Calleman, C. J. (1984). *In* "Biological Monitoring and Surveillance of Workers Exposed to Chemicals" (A. Aitio, V. Riihimaki, and H. Vainio, eds.), pp. 331–337. Hemisphere, Washington, D.C.

Cerutti, P. A. (1985). *Science* **227,** 375–381.

Cerutti, P. *et al.* (1983a). *In* "Extrahepatic Drug Metabolism and Chemical Carcinogenesis" (J. Rydstrom, J. Montelius, and M. Bengtsson, eds.), pp. 449–585. Elsevier, New York.

Cerutti, P. A. *et al.* (1983b). *In* "Genes and Proteins in Oncogenesis" (I. B. Weinstein and H. J. Vogel, eds.), pp. 55–67. Academic Press, New York.

Chambers, J. E., and Yarbrough, J. D. (1982). "Effects of Chronic Exposures to Pesticides on Animal Systems." Raven, New York.

Colburn, N. H. *et al.* (1982). *J. Cell. Biochem.* **18,** 261–270.

Colburn, N. H. *et al.* (1984). *In* "Genes and Cancer" (J. M. Bishop, J. D. Rowley, and M. Greaves, eds.), pp. 137–155. Liss, New York.

Daugaard, J. (1978). "Symptoms and Signs in Occupational Disease, A Practical Guide." Munksgaard, Berlin.

De Serres, F. J., and Ashby, J. (1981). *Prog. Mutat. Res.* **1,** 1–7.

Duesberg, P. H. (1985). *Science* **228,** 669–677.

Dukes, M. N. G., ed. (1980). "Meyler's Side Effects of Drugs," pp. 123–140.

Ehling, U. H. *et al.* (1983). *Mutat. Res.* **123,** 281–341.
Eichler, D. *et al.* (1983). *Xenobiotica* **13,** 639–647.
Emerit, I., and Cerutti, P. (1982). *In* "Mechanisms of Chemical Carcinogenesis" (C. Harris and P. Cerutti, eds.), pp. 495–497. Liss, New York.
Enomoto, T. *et al.* (1981). *Proc. Natl. Acad. Sci. U.S.A.* **78,** 5628–5632.
Farber, E. (1980). *In* "Environmental Chemicals, Enzyme Function and Human Disease" (Ciba Foundation Symposium 76), pp. 261–274. Excerpta Medica, New York.
Fischer, S. (1985). *In* "Arachidonic Acid Metabolism and Tumor Promotion" (S. Fischer and T. J. Slaga, eds.), pp. 255–257. Nijhoff, Boston.
Food Safety Council (1980). "Proposed System for Food Safety Assessment." Washington, D.C.
Fox, T. R., and Watanabe, P. G. (1985). *Science* **228** 596–597.
Frank, H. *et al.* (1982). *Chem. Biol. Interact.* **40,** 193–208.
Gainer, C., and Murray, A. W. (1985). *Biochem. Biophys. Res. Commun.* **126,** 1109–1113.
Gindhart, T. *et al.* (1984). *Carcinogenesis (London)* **5,** 1115–1121.
Griesemer, R. A., and Cueto, C. (1980). *In* "Molecular and Cellular Aspects of Carcinogen Screening Tests" (R. Montesano *et al.*, eds.), pp. 259–281. International Agency for Research on Cancer, Lyon.
Hamm, T. E. (1984). *In* "Mouse Liver Neoplasia" (J. A. Popp, ed.), pp. 27–38. Hemisphere, New York.
Harper, B. L., and Morris, D. L. (1984). *Teratog., Carcinog., Mutagen.* **4,** 483–503.
Harper, B. L. *et al.* (1983). *In* "The Use of Human Cells for the Evaluation of Risk From Physical and Chemical Agents" (A. Castellani, ed.), Vol. 60, pp. 353–424. Plenum, New York.
Haseman, J. K. (1985). *Fundam. Appl. Toxicol.* **5,** 66–78.
Haseman, J. K., *et al.* (1985). *J. Natl. Cancer Inst.* **75,** 975–984.
Hayes, W. T. (1982). "Pesticides Studied in Man." Williams & Wilkins, Baltimore.
Hemminki, K. (1983). *Arch. Toxicol.* **52,** 249–285.
Higginson, J. (1983). *In* "Developments in the Science and Practice of Toxicology" (A. W. Hayes, R. C. Schnell, and T. S. Miya, eds.), pp. 181–190. Elsevier, Amsterdam.
Hirota, F. *et al.* (1984). *Biochem. Biophys. Res. Commun.* **120,** 339–343.
Homa, S. T. *et al.* (1983). *Biochim. Biophys. Acta* **752,** 315–323.
Hooper, K. (1984). *J. Toxicol. Clin. Toxicol.* **22,** 283–289.
Huff, J. E., Melnick, R. L., Solleveld, H. A., Haseman, J. K., Powers, M., and Miller, R. A. (1985). *Science* **227** 548–549.
Hughes, J. P. (1978). *In* "Chemical Hazards of the Workplace" (N. H. Proctor, ed.), pp. 40–54. Lippincott, Philadelphia.
International Agency for Research on Cancer (1979). "Monograph on the Evaluation of the Carcinogenic Risk of Chemicals to Humans. Vol. 20. Some Halogenated Hydrocarbons." IARC, Lyon.
International Commission for Protection Against Environmental Mutagens and Carcinogens (1984). *Mutat. Res.* **133,** 1–49.
Ishidate, K. *et al.* (1982). *Biochim. Biophys Acta* **713,** 103–111.
Josephs, S. F. *et al.* (1984). *Science* **225,** 636–639.
Karenlampis, S. O. *et al.* (1983). *J. Biol. Chem.* **258,** 10378–10383.
Kensler, T. W., and Trush, M. A. (1984). *Environ. Mutagenesis* **6,** 593–616.
Kitagawa, T. *et al.* (1984a). *Proc. Int. Symp. Princess Takamatsu Cancer Res. Fund 1983* (14th Cell Interact. Environ. Tumor Promotors) 337–348.
Kitagawa, T. *et al.* (1984b). *Carcinogenesis* **5,** 1653–1656.
Kliehuis, P. *et al.* (1983). *In* "Developments in the Science and Practice of Toxicology" (A. W. Hayes, R. C. Schnell, and T. S. Miya, eds.), pp. 255–264. Elsevier, Amsterdam.
Kris, R. M. *et al.* (1985). *Biotechnology* **Feb.** 135–140.

Kunz, H. W., Tennekes, H. A., Port, R. E., Schwartz, M., Lorke, D., and Schaude, G. (1983). *Environ. Health Perspect.* **50,** 113–122.

Lamb, R. G., and Schwertz, D. W. (1982). *Toxicol. Appl. Pharmacol.* **63,** 216–229.

Larsson, L. G. (1984). Annu. Meet. Eur. Soc. Ther. Radiol. Oncol., 3rd Sept. 9–15.

Lawley, P. D. (1979). *In* "Chemical Carcinogens and DNA" (P. L. Grover, ed.), Vol. I, pp. 1–36. CRC Press, Boca Raton, Florida.

Leonard, T. B., Dent, J. G., and Graichen, M. E. (1983). *Proc. Am. Assoc. Cancer Res.* **24,** 221.

McPhail, L. C. *et al.* (1984). *Science* **224,** 622–625.

Marx, J. L. (1985). *Science* **228,** 312–313.

Mitchell, J. R. *et al.* (1984). *In* "Drug Metabolism and Drug Toxicity" (J. R. Mitchell and M. G. Horning, eds.), pp. 301–319. Raven, New York.

Morgan, K. T. *et al.* (1984). *J. Natl. Cancer Inst.* **72,** 151–160.

Murphree, A. L., and Benedict, W. F. (1984). *Science* **223,** 1028–1033.

National Toxicology Program (1984). Report of the NTP Ad Hoc Panel on Chemical Carcinogenesis Testing and Evaluation. Washington, D.C.

Newberne, P. M. (1982). *In* "Free Radicals, Lipid Peroxidation and Cancer" (D. C. H. McBrien and T. F. Slater, eds.), pp. 243–290. Academic Press, London.

Nishizuka, Y. (1984a). *Nature (London)* **308** 693–698.

Nishizuka, Y. (1984b). *Science* **225,** 1365–1370.

Parke, D. V., and Ioannides, C. (1984). *In* "Mechanisms of Hepatocyte Injury and Death" (D. Keppler, H. Popper, L. Bianchi, and W. Reutter, eds.), 38th Falk Symposium, pp. 37–48. MTP Press, Lancaster.

Peraino, C. *et al.* (1983). *In* "Mechanisms of Tumor Promotion" (T. J. Slaga, ed.), pp. 1–53. CRC Press, Boca Raton, Florida.

Perera, F. P. (1984). *Environ. Res.* **34,** 175–191.

Pitot, H. C., and Sirica, A. E. (1980). *Biochim. Biophys. Acta* **605,** 191–215.

Popp, James A. *et al.* (1984). "Mouse Liver Neoplasia: Current Perspectives." Hemisphere, Washington, D.C.

Popp, J. A. *et al.* (1985). *Fundam. Appl. Toxicol.* **5,** 314–319.

Popper, H. (1984). *In* "Mechanisms of Hepatocyte Injury and Death" (D. Keppler *et al.* eds.), pp. 37–48. MTP Press, Lancaster.

Ramel, C. (1984). *Acta Pharmacol. Toxicol. (Copenhagen)* **55** (Suppl 2), 181–196.

Reddy, J. K. *et al.* (1983). *Toxicol. Pathol.* **11,** 172–180.

Reitz, R. H., and Watanabe, P. G. (1983). *In* "Developments in the Science and Practice of Toxicology" (A. W. Hayes, R. C. Schnell, and T. S. Miya, eds.), pp. 163–172. Elsevier, Amsterdam.

Reynolds, E. S., and Moslen, M. T. (1980). *In* "Toxic Injury of the Liver, Part B" (E. Farber and M. M. Fisher, eds.), pp. 541–596. Dekker, New York.

Rinkus, S. J., and Legator, M. S. (1980). *Chem. Mutagens* **6,** 365–473.

Schulte-Hermann, R., Schuppler, J., Timmermann-Trosiener, I., Ohde, G., Bursch, W., and Berger, H. (1983a). *Environ. Health Perspect.* **50,** 185–194.

Schulte-Hermann, R., Timmermann-Trosiener, I., and Schuppler, J. (1983b). *Cancer Res.* **43,** 839–844.

Schwarz, M. *et al.* (1984). *Carcinogenesis (London)* **5,** 1663–1670.

Sittig, M. (1981). "Handbook of Toxic and Hazardous Chemicals." Noyes, Park Ridge, New Jersey.

Slaga, T. J. (1983). *Environ. Health Perspect.* **50,** 3–14.

Slaga, T. J., and Digiovanni, J. (1984). *In* "Inhibition of Chemical Carcinogenesis" (Charles E. Searle, ed.), Vol. II, pp. 1279–1321. American Chemical Society, Washington, D.C.

Slaga, T. J., and Fischer, S. (1985). *In* "Arachidonic Acid Metabolism and Tumor Promotion" (S. M. Fisher and T. J. Slaga, eds.), pp. 255–257. Nijhoff, Boston.
Sobels, F. H. (1984). *Mutat. Res.* **130,** 425–428.
Stevens, F. J., and Peraino, C. (1983). *In* "Organ and Species Specificity in Chemical Carcinogenesis" (R. Langenbach and S. Nesnow, eds.), pp. 231–252. Plenum, New York.
Sukumar, S. *et al.* (1984). *Science* **223,** 1197–1199.
Swenson, D. H. (1983). *In* "Developments in the Science and Practice of Toxicology" (A. W. Hayes, R. C. Schnell, and T. S. Miya, eds.), pp. 247–254. Elsevier, Amsterdam.
Tainsky, M. A. *et al.* (1984). *Science* **225,** 643–645.
Tarone, R. E. *et al.* (1981). *J. Natl. Cancer Inst.* **66,** 1175–1181.
Tewey, K. M. *et al.* (1984). *Science* **225,** 466–468.
Tomasi, A. *et al.* (1984). *Toxicol. Pathol.* **12,** 240–246.
Trosko, J. E., and Chang, C. C. (1981). *Adv. Radiat. Biol.* **9,** 1–36.
Trosko, J. E. *et al.* (1982). *Carcinogenesis* **3,** 1101–1103.
Tsushimoto, G. *et al.* (1983. *Arch. Environ. Contam. Toxicol.* **12,** 721–730.
U.S. Environmental Protection Agency Office of Toxic Substances (1982). Health Effects Test Guidelines and Support Documents.
Varmus, H. E. (1984). *Environ. Sci. Res.* **31,** 61–77.
Vesselinovitch, S. D. *et al.* (1977). *Cancer Res.* **37,** 1822–1828.
Walder, L., and Lutzelschwab, R. (1984). *Exp. Cell Res.* **152,** 66–76.
Ward, J. B. *et al.* (1981). *In* "Microbial Testers" (I. C. Felkner, ed.), Vol. 5, pp. 167–186. Dekker, New York.
Ward, J. M. (1984). *In* "Mouse Liver Neoplasia" (J. A. Popp, ed.), pp. 1–26. Hemisphere, New York.
Ward, J. M. *et al.* (1979). *J. Natl. Cancer Inst.* **63,** 849–854.
Wechsler, W. *et al.* (1979). *Natl. Cancer Inst. Monogr.* **51,** 219–226.
Weinstein, I. B. (1981). *J. Supramol. Struct. Cell. Biochem.* **17,** 99–120.
Weisburger, J. H., and Williams, G. M. (1981). *Science* **211,** 401–407.
Weisburger, J. H., and Williams, G. M. (1983). *Environ. Health Perspect.* **50,** 233–245.
Weisburger, J. H., and Wynder, E. L. (1984). *Acta Pharmacol. Toxicol. (Copenhagen)* **55** (Suppl 2), 53–68.
Williams, G. M. (1983a). *Environ. Health Perspect.* **50,** 177–183.
Williams, G. M. (1983b). *Ann. N.Y. Acad. Sci.* **407,** 328–333.
Willson, R. L. (1982). *In* "Free Radicals, Lipid Peroxidation and Cancer" (D. C. H. McBrien and T. F. Slater, eds.), pp. 275–302. Academic Press, London.
Wiman, K. G., Clarkson, B., Hayday, A. C., Saito, H., Tonegawa, S., and Hayward, W. S. (1984). *Proc. Natl. Acad. Sci. U.S.A.* **81,** 6798–6802.
Yamasaki, H. (1984). *Acta Pharmacol. Toxicol. (Copenhagen)* **55** (Suppl 2), 89–106.
Yunis, J. J., and Soreng, A. L. (1984). *Science* **226,** 1199–1204.
Yuspa, S. H. (1983). *In* "Extrahepatic Drug Metabolism and Chemical Carcinogenesis" (J. Rydstrom, J. Montelius, and M. Bengtsson, eds.), pp. 547–556. Elsevier, New York.
Yu-Yan, Z., and Zhen, Y. (1985). *In* "Subclinical Hepatocellular Carcinoma" (Z.-Y. Tang, ed.), pp. 298–320. Springer-Verlag, Berlin.
Zeiger, E., and Tennant, R. W. (1985). 4th *Int. Conf. Environ. Mutagens, Stockholm, June.*
Zimmermann, F. K. *et al.* (1985). *Mutat. Res.* **150,** 203–210.
Zimmermann, H. J. (1980). *In* "Toxic Injury of the Liver, Part B" (E. Farber and M. M. Fisher, eds.), pp. 687–737. Dekker, New York.
Zimmermann, H. J. (1982). *In* "Toxicology of the Liver" (G. Plaa and W. R. Hewitt, eds.), pp. 1–45. Raven, New York.

ADVANCES IN VETERINARY SCIENCE AND COMPARATIVE MEDICINE, VOL. 31

The Significance of Preneoplastic Liver Lesions in Experimental Animals

GARY M. WILLIAMS

Naylor Dana Institute for Disease Prevention, American Health Foundation, Valhalla, New York 10595

I. Introduction

During the experimental induction of liver cancer in rodents, several distinct cellular lesions precede the development of malignant neoplasms. Among those that have been postulated to be precursors of hepatocellular cancer are "oval cell" proliferation (Farber, 1956; Inaoka, 1967), altered (hyperplastic) foci (Firminger, 1955; Reuber, 1965; Newberne and Wogan, 1968; Bannasch, 1968; Friedrich-Freksa *et al.*, 1969), and hyperplastic (neoplastic) nodules (Firminger, 1955; Reuber, 1965; Newberne and Wogan, 1968; Farber, 1973).

Oval cells can appear in rat liver within days of administration of a hepatocarcinogen. They are small oval cells, as their name indicates, with scant cytoplasms and pale nuclei. They are usually concentrated in the periportal regions and have generally been thought to be of bile ductular origin (Grisham and Porta, 1964; Rubin, 1964). The finding of some hepatocellular properties in these cells has been interpreted as evidence that they may be related to hepatocytes, possibly as stem cells (Sell *et al.*, 1981), although this must be taken cautiously because of the possibility of aberrant gene expression in the oval cells.

The altered focus is the earliest-appearing distinct lesion of hepatocytes induced by liver carcinogens. Foci, as described in several species, are lesions smaller than a lobule and are composed of cells with abnormal staining properties and a variety of phenotypic abnormalities. Usually, the cells are different in size from hepatocytes and display nuclear abnormalities. The cells of foci are usually organized in plates which merge with those of the surrounding normal parenchyma. Ultrastructural studies have revealed distinct hepatocellular characteristics of the cells in foci (Timme, 1978; Hirota *et al.*, 1982).

Nodular lesions that have been designated as hyperplastic or neoplastic appear later in carcinogenesis than foci. Nodules are composed of cells similar to those in foci, but they are larger and compress the surrounding parenchyma from which they are sharply demarcated. Cells in nodules possess many of the ultrastructural properties of hepatocytes (Farber, 1973).

II. Significance of Preneoplastic Lesions

The term "preneoplastic" has been given various meanings. In the present context, it will be used to designate cellular populations that precede the development of neoplasms and from which neoplasms apparently evolve. Within such populations some cells may already be neoplastic, but at present, there is no means to identify these.

A. Oval Cells

Oval cell proliferation is prominent in the early stages of hepatocarcinogenesis in rat liver with several different carcinogens, particularly aminoazo dyes and aromatic amines (Farber, 1956; Inaoka, 1967; Dempo *et al.*, 1975; Guillouzo *et al.*, 1981), and under conditions of lipotrope deficiency (Shinozuka *et al.*, 1978), which can enhance or even by itself lead to liver cancer. Consequently, oval cells have been suggested to be progenitors of liver neoplasms. However, they do not occur regularly with administration of all hepatocarcinogens (Williams and Yamamato, 1972) and are induced by noncarcinogenic treatments (Lopez and Mazzanti, 1955; Grisham and Hartroft, 1961). Moreover, oval cells have not been documented in mouse or hamster liver. Therefore, their value and significance as a general indicator of hepatocarcinogenesis is not well established.

B. Altered Foci

Most studies of the pathogenesis of foci have been done in rat liver. Foci are rapidly induced in rat liver by hepatocarcinogens, and they also appear spontaneously in older rats (Ogawa *et al.*, 1981; Ward, 1981). The numbers of induced foci are related to the dose of carcinogen (Emmelot and Scherer, 1980). They increase in number and size with continued carcinogen exposure (Williams and Watanabe, 1978; Rabes and Szymkowiak, 1979) or with time after cessation of certain carcinogen exposures (Barbason and Betz, 1981; Moore *et al.*, 1981). After some conditions of carcinogen exposure, certain phenotypic abnormalities in foci are quite persistent and stable (Pitot *et al.*, 1978). Under other conditions, after cessation of carcinogen exposure, the expression of some phenotypic abnormalities in foci can diminish, a phenomenon referred to as phenotypic reversion (Williams and Watanabe, 1978). Whether the cells in reverting or regressing foci actually are lost, as suggested by some studies (Bursch *et al.*, 1984), or whether they persist in a latent state (Williams, 1980), remains to be resolved.

Rat liver foci apparently develop by the clonal expansion of an altered cell (Rabes *et al.*, 1982). Their growth rate has been related to the complexity of phenotypic abnormalities in their cells (Pitot *et al.*, 1978; Pugh and Goldfarb, 1978; Peraino *et al.*, 1984). As a result of sustained growth, foci develop into nodular lesions (Williams, 1976). For those who believe that nodules are hyperplastic (see below) and are the direct precursors of carcinomas, foci would not be considered preneoplastic. For those who believe that nodules are neoplasms, foci would be considered preneoplastic.

One proposal concerning the biological behavior of foci is that they have the potential to develop into either nodules (adenomas) or carcinomas (Williams, 1980). In support of this suggestion, microspectrophotometric study of the DNA content of cells in foci, nodules, and carcinomas revealed that eosinophilic foci and nodules both had a wide range of DNA contents whereas hyperbasophilic foci had an aneuploid DNA content like carcinomas (Mori *et al.*, 1982a). It is possible, therefore, that eosinophilic foci may develop into nodules and basophilic foci into carcinomas. Studies of transplantation of foci have not revealed progressive growth (Mori *et al.*, 1983) and, thus, there is no evidence that foci are neoplastic.

The development of carcinomas from foci may require further genetic alterations in the cells of foci. Recently, evidence has been provided that cells in rat liver foci have a lesser DNA repair capacity than normal cells (Mori *et al.*, 1985a). This could make them more susceptible to genetic alteration during continued carcinogen exposure, even though they are less susceptible to toxic effects of activation-dependent carcinogens (Williams *et al.*, 1976) as a consequence of reduced carcinogen activation and increased detoxification systems (Okita *et al.*, 1976; Judah *et al.*, 1977; Kuhlmann *et al.*, 1981; Astrom *et al.*, 1983; Kitahara *et al.*, 1983).

Clearly, only a small fraction of foci develop into neoplasms, since foci greatly outnumber neoplasms (Reuber, 1965; Rabes *et al.,* 1972; Scherer *et al.,* 1972; Williams *et al.,* 1976; Williams and Watanabe, 1978; Barbason and Betz. 1981; Takahashi *et al.,* 1982). Estimates of the rate of progression are in the order of 1 in 1000 (Watanabe and Williams, 1978) to 1 in 2500 (Pitot *et al.,* 1978). Probably, different types of foci have different potentials for developing into neoplasms.

The demonstration that the progression of foci to neoplasm formation is enhanced by promoters (Pitot *et al.,* 1978; Kitagawa and Sugano, 1978; Watanabe and Williams, 1978) provides further evidence that they are a source of neoplasms. Nevertheless, observations that they can remain dormant or even undergo phenotypic reversion indicates that they are not committed to neoplastic development, but may be truly preneoplastic.

C. Adenomas

Nodules usually develop at a later stage of carcinogenesis, after induction of foci (Reuber, 1965; Williams and Yamamato, 1972). Their nature is controversial. For many years, they have been considered to be hyperplastic and to be precursors of carcinomas (Firminger, 1955; Reuber, 1965; Newberne *et al.,* 1968; Farber, 1973). Support for the view that rat nodules are hyperplastic comes mainly from studies in which nodules have been reported to disappear following cessation of carcinogen exposure (Teebor and Becker, 1971). Recent experiments concerned with this possibility involve cytotoxic selection of lesions induced very early in carcinogenesis (Ogawa *et al.,* 1980; Tatematsu *et al.,* 1980). Without such a selective pressure, the lesions involved would probably be regarded as altered foci rather than nodules, and, therefore, the behavior of this type of nodular lesion can be interpreted as representing a special situation in which foci have become nodular because of rapid growth. As would then be expected, nodules of this type behave similarly to foci in their high frequency of phenotypic reversion.

The nature of nodules that are produced under conventional modalities of chronic exposure or that arise after cessation of carcinogen exposure is apparently different. Such nodules in rats are persistent and progressively growing (Hirota and Williams, 1979a). The growth capability of nodules, however, is apparently limited, since they have not displayed progressive growth in transplantation studies (Williams *et al.,* 1977, 1980), even when recipients were treated with phenobarbital (Mori *et al.,* 1983). Nevertheless, Wanson *et al.* (1981) reported that when nodule fragments were brought into contact with precultured embryonic chick heart fragments, they invaded the heart tissue, suggesting that some nodule cells are even malignant.

Several expert groups have now recommended that rat nodules be designated as neoplastic (Squire and Levitt, 1975; Stewart *et al.*, 1980). This is based in part on the fact that typical-appearing nodules can give rise to metastases, indicating that they are malignant.

The nature of mouse liver nodules has been equally controversial (see Butler and Newberne, 1975; Doull *et al.*, 1983). To reflect the uncertainty about the nature of nodular lesions, in early studies well-differentiated nodules were designated as "type A," while those with cellular dysplasia were referred to as "type B." There is now a general consensus that type B nodules are carcinomas. Type A nodules were shown by Williams *et al.* (1979) to be transplantable. Moreover, they have many of the same phenotypic alterations as carcinomas (Numoto *et al.*, 1985a). In consideration of these observations, it seems appropriate to designate such nodules as adenomas.

Thus, nodules in both rat and mouse liver can be regarded as neoplastic rather than preneoplastic lesions and referred to as adenomas.

In summary, it appears that there are several possible pathways for the development of liver cancer. One of these involves the altered focus as a significant "preneoplastic" population. The remainder of this review will describe studies on the characteristics of foci and the use of quantitation of foci to monitor effects of chemicals on liver carcinogenesis.

III. Characteristics of Altered Foci

A. Rat

Based upon abnormalities in the H and E staining properties of the cells in rat foci, they can be classified as eosinophilic (Fig. 1), basophilic (Fig. 2), or clear (Fig. 3). Mixed types also occur.

A variety of other phenotypic abnormalities have been identified in altered foci (Table I). The expression of these varies in the different types of foci and among foci of each type.

1. *Enzyme Histochemical Markers*

Foci have been demonstrated to display a variety of enzyme abnormalities such as reduced activity of glucose-6-phosphatase (G-6-Pase) (Gössner and Friedrich-Freksa, 1964; Bannasch, 1968) and adenosine triphosphatase (ATPase) (Kitagawa, 1971; Rabes *et al.*, 1972; Scherer

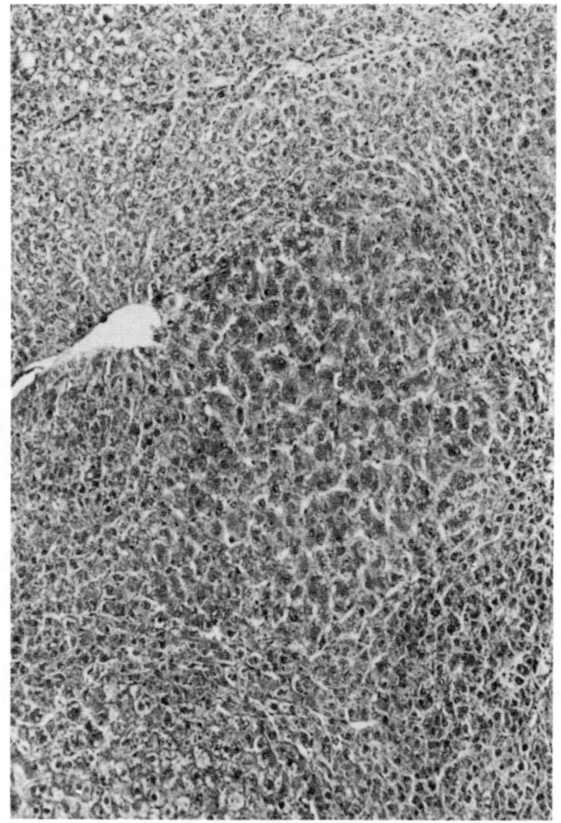

FIG. 1. Rat liver eosinophilic altered focus. Hematoxylin and eosin; ×112.

et al., 1972), and reappearance of γ-glutamyl transpeptidase (GGT) activity (Kalengayi *et al.,* 1975; Harada *et al.,* 1976). The latter is a fetal liver enzyme that diminishes to low levels of activity in adult liver but is elevated in liver tumors (Fiala *et al.,* 1976). Also, the appearance of abnormal enzymes such as aldehyde dehydrogenase (Jones *et al.,* 1984) and a placental form of glutathione transferase (Kitahara *et al.,* 1984) has been described. All these properties are generally uniform in their expression within a focus, but distinctly heterogeneous between different foci (Pitot *et al.,* 1978; Kitagawa, 1971; Pugh and Goldfarb, 1978; Hirota and Williams, 1979b).

Importantly, histochemical markers can be used on biopsy samples obtained by fine-needle aspiration of the rat liver (Boelsterli and

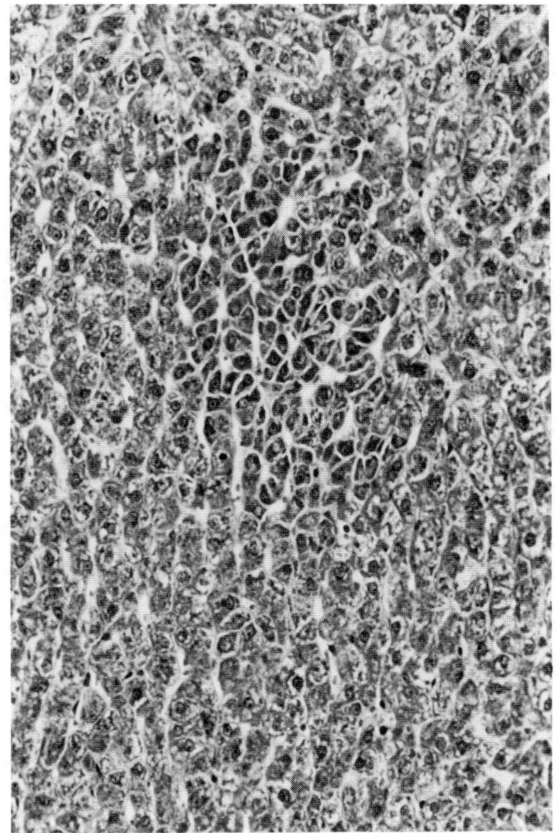

FIG. 2. Rat liver basophilic cell altered focus. Hematoxylin and eosin; ×45.

Zbinden, 1979), permitting individual animals to be followed by serial punctures over a long time period. Moreover, serum GGT is elevated in rats exposed to either a hepatocarcinogen or a liver tumor promoter (Remandet *et al.,* 1984) and, therefore, can be used as an index of hepatocarcinogenesis.

2. *Glycogen*

Bannasch (1968) first reported that nitrosamine-induced foci displayed excessive storage of glycogen. Subsequently, glycogen-storing foci were demonstrated with other types of carcinogens (Williams *et*

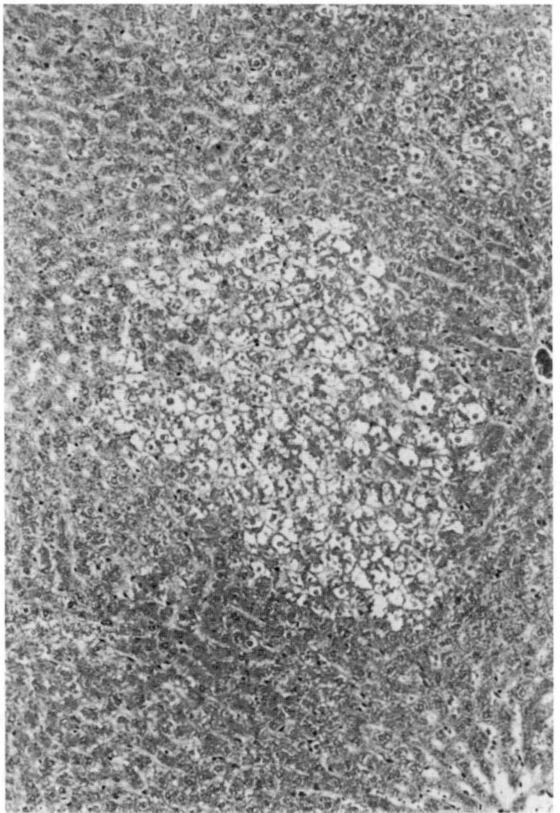

FIG. 3. Rat liver clear cell altered focus. Hematoxylin and eosin; ×112.

al., 1976). This abnormality appears to be related at least in part to a deficiency of G-6-Pase in foci cells.

3. *Exclusion of Cellular Iron*

A deficiency in the accumulation of cellular iron during either dietary or parenteral iron overload was shown by Williams and associates (Williams and Yamamoto, 1972; Williams, 1976; Williams *et al.,* 1979) to characterize cells in foci, nodules, and carcinomas in rat liver. This property provides a highly sensitive marker for the detection of altered foci during carcinogen administration, permitting quantitative studies of hepatocarcinogenesis (Williams and Watanabe, 1978; Hirota and Williams, 1979a; Malvaldi, 1981). Following discontinua-

TABLE I

PHENOTYPIC ABNORMALITIES OF HEPATOCELLULAR ALTERED FOCI

Enzymes
Deficiency glucose-6-phosphatase
Deficiency adenosine triphosphatase
Increased γ-glutamyl transpeptidase
Increased placental form of glutathione transferase
Appearance of aldehyde dehydrogenase
Excessive glycogen storage
Exclusion of cellular iron
Resistance to cytotoxic effects of toxins requiring metabolism

tion of exposure, a phenotypic reversion of this property can occur whereby the cells in foci reacquire the ability to store cellular iron (Williams and Watanabe, 1978; Furuya *et al.,* 1984).

As a marker, exclusion of iron has a number of advantages. It is applicable to all species studied thus far (see below). Also, the ability to distinguish between iron-excluding and iron-engorged cells at the ultrastructural level has facilitated reliable electron-microscopic studies of ultrastructural abnormalities in altered foci (Timme, 1978; Hirota and Williams, 1982). Iron exclusion is the only marker that results in a difference in the density of altered cells rendering them separable on density gradients (Mori *et al.,* 1982b).

GGT activity and ATPase deficiency appear to be quite persistent in foci following cessation of carcinogen exposure. However, care is required in the use of GGT as a marker because activity can be induced in periportal hepatocytes by xenobiotics (Furukawa *et al.,* 1984), which also induce drug-metabolizing enzymes, and activity is elevated in aged rats, particularly females.

4. *α-Fetoprotein Production*

In 1963, Abelev made the discovery of the appearance of a fetal protein, α-fetoprotein (AFP), in the serum of adult mice with liver cancer (Abelev, 1971). Subsequently, production of this protein by both human and rat hepatocellular carcinomas was documented. Moreover, several laboratories (Watabe, 1971; Kitagawa *et al.,* 1972; Kroes *et al.,* 1972) independently found that an increase in serum AFP could be detected within a few weeks of carcinogen administration, long before the development of liver cancers. After early induction, if carcinogen exposure was discontinued, AFP diminished and reappeared only with the development of liver neoplasms. Thus, elevation of serum AFP was established as a indicator both of the early effects of liver carcinogens and of the presence of liver neoplasms.

The basis for the appearance of serum AFP early in hepatocarcinogenesis has been somewhat controversial. In several of the studies that first documented this phenomenon, AFP was associated with the proliferation of oval cells (Watabe, 1971; Kroes *et al.,* 1973; Dempo *et al.,* 1975). Subsequently, immunofluorescent and immunoperoxidase staining confirmed the localization of AFP to these cells, but not those in foci (Tchipysheva *et al.,* 1977; Kuhlmann, 1978; Sell, 1978; Guillouzo *et al.,* 1981). Another possibility for early AFP production suggested by Kroes *et al.* (1972) was the direct or indirect derepression by hepatocarcinogens of the gene or genes responsible for AFP production.

Thus, several mechanisms may exist for elevated AFP levels early in hepatocarcinogenesis. Although cellular localization of AFP is apparently not a useful marker for foci, elevated serum levels may be used as an indicator of hepatocarcinogenesis and is one of the few properties that can also be monitored in humans.

5. *Resistance to Cytotoxicity*

The resistance of neoplastic cells to the cytotoxic effects of carcinogens was documented by Haddow (1938) and expanded by later investigators, in particular Vasiliev and Guelstein (1963). Farber and co-workers demonstrated that altered foci (Williams *et al.,* 1976) and hyperplastic nodules (Farber *et al.,* 1979) in rat liver were similarly resistant to cytotoxicity. The resistance appears to result largely from reduced xenobiotic activation and enhanced detoxification systems (Okita *et al.,* 1976; Judah *et al.,* 1977; Kuhlmann *et al.,* 1981; Astrom *et al.,* 1983; Kitahara *et al.,* 1983). As a result of greater activation of carcinogens by normal liver cells, an antimiotic effect is exerted on them and, consequently, they are impaired in responding to a mitogenic stimulus such as partial hepatectomy, whereas proliferation occurs in altered foci and nodules. By this means foci can be rendered more conspicuous for detection in bioassay of carcinogens (Farber, 1979).

B. Mouse

Foci in mouse liver are not as conspicuous as in the rat. The best recognized type of focus is that composed of basophilic cells (Fig. 4).

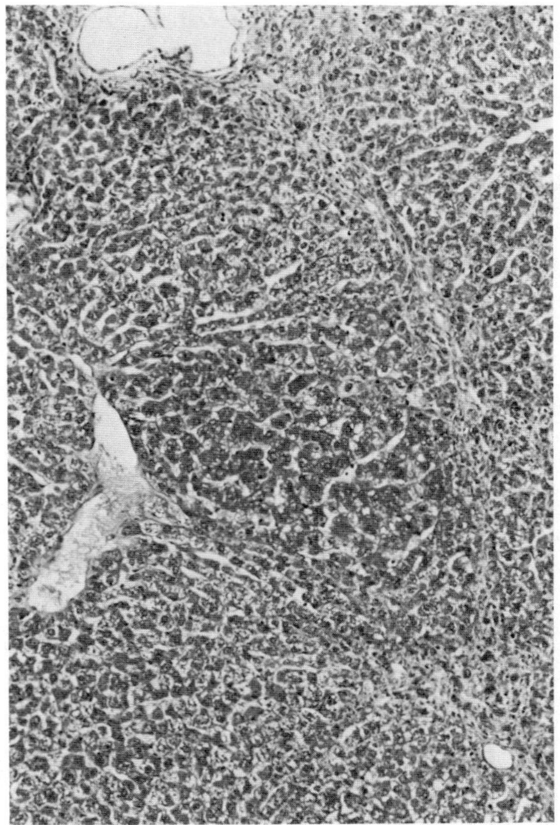

FIG. 4. Mouse liver basophilic altered focus. Hematoxylin and eosin; ×99.

Mouse foci also display a variety of phenotypic abnormalities, but these are more variable than in the rat (Lipsky *et al.*, 1980; Ohmori *et al.*, 1981). Among enzyme histochemical markers, G-6-Pase and GGT appear to be reliable (Lipsky *et al.*, 1980; Moore *et al.*, 1981; Cater *et al.*, 1985). Iron exclusion is also a fairly consistent property (Williams *et al.*, 1979; Cater *et al.*, 1985).

C. HAMSTER

Only a single study of foci in hamster livers has been reported (Stenbäck *et al.*, 1986). Foci induced by dimethylnitrosamine were composed mainly of clear cells (Fig. 5) and were iron-excluding, but not GGT-positive.

D. Monkey

Administration of diethylnitrosamine by i.p. injection to male rhesus monkeys induced foci by 6 months (Ruebner *et al.*, 1976). The foci were composed of cells with clear cytoplasms due to large amounts of glycogen storage. Foci also displayed decreased G-6-Pase activity and a change in the distribution of ATPase.

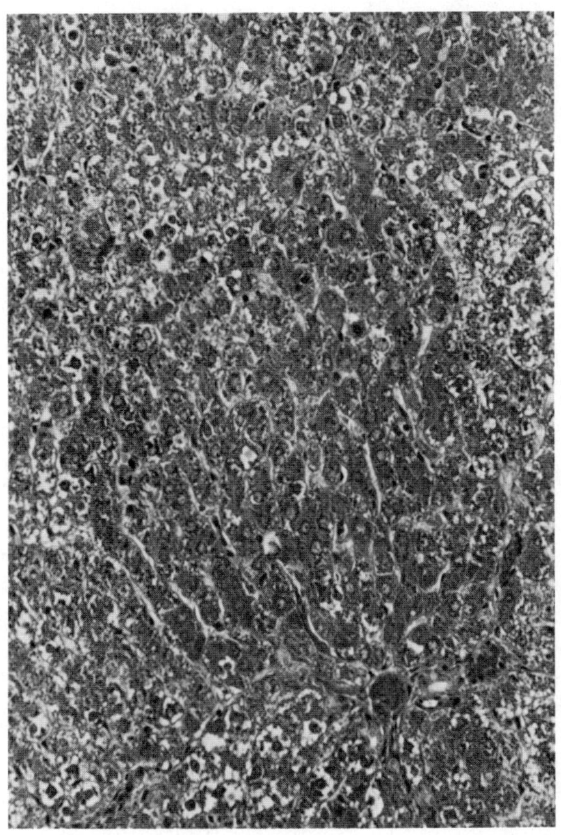

Fig. 5. Hamster liver altered focus. Hematoxylin and eosin; ×257.

IV. Induction of Altered Foci as a Means of Detecting Carcinogens

Because foci are induced in the livers of several species by carcinogens and because of the evidence that they are related to the development of liver neoplasms (i.e., are preneoplastic), the induction of foci has been proposed as one type of limited *in vivo* bioassay for detecting carcinogens (Weisburger and Williams, 1981; Pereira, 1982).

In the application of this approach, it must be recognized that chemicals defined operationally as carcinogens by the production of neoplasms after chronic administration, include both agents which are DNA-reactive and consequently capable of inducing neoplastic conversion and others which are not DNA-reactive, but exert effects on neoplastic development that result in enhanced tumor formation. Therefore, Weisburger and Williams (1980) have proposed the classification of carcinogens into two major categories, genotoxic and epigenetic. This concept is discussed elsewhere in this monograph (see Ashby). Genotoxic carcinogens are defined as those capable of reacting with DNA. The capacity of chemicals to damage DNA has been established to be closely related to their carcinogenicity and probably is the basis for this biological effect.

The rapid induction of foci is an action of genotoxic hepatocarcinogens, occasionally resulting from a single exposure, but usually occurring in less than 12 weeks and increasing with continued administration. Therefore, examination of the liver for foci at 8–12 weeks of continued or repeated administration of a test compound is a reasonable limited bioassay for genotoxic carcinogens. In fact, even carcinogens that may be only weakly or indirectly genotoxic such as methapyrilene can be detected by this approach (Furuya and Williams, 1984).

In assaying for foci induction, some investigators have advocated the use of only a single exposure, usually in conjunction with phenobarbital (Pereira, 1982) or some other form of enhancement such as partial hepatectomy (Pitot and Sirica, 1980) or feeding of a choline-deficient diet (Shinozuka *et al.*, 1979). The rapid induction of "nodules" has been described using partial hepatectomy combined with administration of 2-acetylaminofluorene (Tatematsu *et al.*, 1977; Tsuda *et al.*, 1980). Such complex procedures have not been shown to be essential for the detection of any carcinogen and entail two problems. Although such procedures may enhance the development of carcinogen-induced lesions, chemicals that are positive under conditions of combined exposures or treatments can only be regarded as *suspect* carcinogens, since carcinogens are defined by their effects in the absence of deliberate exposure to any other agents. On the other hand, negative results in such assays are of very limited value because measurement of induction of lesions with a single or few exposures may simply lack sufficient sensitivity. In contrast, continuous administration either in feed, by gavage, or by injection for at least 8–12 weeks provides a more rigorous and interpretable assay for carcinogenicity. This can be followed by phenobarbital to enhance sensitivity further.

Some of the agents that have been tested under appropriate conditions are listed in Table II. Chemicals that were negative in assays using single or limited exposures are not tabulated, since these results are not of great strength. It is evident from the results in Table II that a wide variety of structurally different carcinogens can be identified by the production of altered liver foci during limited exposure.

V. Enhancement of Altered Foci as a Means of Identifying Neoplasm-Promoting Agents

The demonstration that the liver neoplasm promoter phenobarbital enhanced the persistence and progression of altered foci in rat liver (Kitagawa *et al.,* 1978; Pitot *et al.,* 1978; Watanabe and Williams, 1978) provided the basis for an approach to the rapid detection of liver neoplasm promoters. In the subsequent applications of this phenomenon, the general approach has been to administer a genotoxic hepatocarcinogen first and then to give the test agent to determine if it has an enhancing effect upon the number or size of foci (Williams, 1982). Studies have also been made of increased DNA synthesis in foci (Schulte-Hermann *et al.,* 1981).

In measuring the enhancement of foci as evidence of promotion, it must be remembered that two genotoxic liver carcinogens administered sequentially will produce a summation effect, which results in an increase in foci (Williams *et al.,* 1981). This phenomenon, which also occurs when two carcinogens are administered together (Mori *et al.,* 1985b), results in syncarcinogenesis, which must be distinguished from promotion (Williams and Furuya, 1984; Kuchlbauer *et al.,* 1985). Therefore, in studying the enhancement of foci as evidence of neoplasm promotion, it is essential that the test agent first should be demonstrated to be nongenotoxic and to produce an enhancement only when given after and not before a genotoxic carcinogen. Thus far, only

TABLE II

EFFECT OF CHEMICALS STUDIED FOR PRODUCTION OF ALTERED FOCI IN RODENT LIVER

Chemical	Species	Effect[a]	References
Acetaminophen	Rat	−	Tsuda *et al.* (1984)
Aflatoxin B_1	Rat	+	Kalengayi *et al.* (1975)
Aminoazo dyes			
4-Dimethylaminoazobenzene	Rat	+	Timme (1978)
3′-Methyl-4-(dimethyl-amino)-azobenzene	Rat	+	Tatematsu *et al.* (1983)
Auramine	Rat	w	Tatematsu *et al.* (1983)
Butylated hdyroxyanisole	Rat	−	Tsuda *et al.* (1984)
Benzodiazepines			
Clorazepate	Rat	−	Mazue *et al.* (1982)
Diazapam	Rat	−	Mazue *et al.* (1982)
Lorazepam	Rat	−	Mazue *et al.* (1982)
Oxazepam	Rat	−	Mazue *et al.* (1982)
Dimethylhydrazine	Rat	+	Herren *et al.* (1982)
Ethoxyquin	Rat	−	Tsuda *et al.* (1984)
Methapyrilene	Rat	+	Furuya and Williams (1984)
Nitrosamines	Rat	+	Williams and Yamamoto (1972)
Diethylnitrosamine	Rat	+	Scherer *et al.* (1972)
	Mouse	+	Peraino *et al.* (1981)
Dimethylnitrosamine	Rat	+	Herren *et al.* (1982)
	Hamster	+	Stenbäck *et al.* (1986)
N-Ethyl-*N*-hydroxyethyl nitrosamine	Rat	+	Tsuda *et al.* (1984)
Polycyclic aromatic hydrocarbons			
Benz[*a*]anthracene	Rat	+	Tsuda *et al.* (1980)
Benzo[*a*]pyrene	Rat	+	Peraino *et al.* (1981)
	Mouse	+	Peraino *et al.* (1981)
Pyrolysate products			
Trp-P-1	Rat	+	Ishikawa *et al.* (1979)
Trp-P-2	Rat	+/−	Ishikawa *et al.* (1979)
Safrole	Mouse	+	Lipsky *et al.* (1980)
Trichloroethylene	Rat	−	Laib *et al.* (1979)
Urethane	Rat	+	Herren *et al.* (1982)
Vinyl bromide	Rat	+	Bolt *et al.* (1979)
Vinyl chloride	Rat	+	Laib *et al.* (1979)

[a] −, Negative; +, positive; w, weak positive.

phenobarbital has been shown to fulfill these requirements (Schwarz *et al.,* 1983; Williams and Furuya, 1984). Unfortunately, enhancement of foci by genotoxic agents is often uncritically reported as promotion (Reilly *et al.,* 1985; Shirai *et al.,* 1985).

An important extension of these concepts is that the absence of an enhancing effect of a compound administered after a genotoxic carcinogen indicates an absence of summation and therefore provides evidence of a lack of genotoxicity (Williams, 1984).

The general approach of administering a genotoxic carcinogen followed by a second agent to test for promotion has many variations (Leonard *et al.,* 1982; Williams, 1982). Some involve a powerful initial carcinogenic exposure, such as diethylnitrosamine plus partial hepatectomy, while others involve intense combination effects such as with the feeding of 2-acetylaminofluorene coupled with partial hepatectomy. The model developed by Williams differs from these in several respects. In this model, a genotoxic carcinogen, usually 2-acetylaminofluorene, is administered in the diet in the first phase for 8–12 weeks. This results in the gradual induction of foci such that at the time of administration of the second agent after an interval of cessation of exposure of 2–4 weeks, foci are already present. The main purpose of this is to distinguish promotion from cocarcinogenic effects. Promotion, by definition (Berenblum, 1974), involves facilitation of the growth of neoplastic cells. By first inducing detectable foci, the effect of the second agent on a carcinogen-altered population, which probably includes neoplastic cells (see Section II,B), is demonstrated. In regimens where a carcinogen is followed shortly by a second agent, before foci appear, enhancement can be due to increased neoplastic conversion of carcinogen-damaged cells, which is really a cocarcinogenic effect (Williams, 1984). It is also for this reason that an interval of 2–4 weeks is allowed between administration of the initiating carcinogen and commencement of exposure to the second agent. Other reasons for the protracted initiation phase are to standardize a model for the reliable detection of genotoxic carcinogens (Section IV) and to have a model in which the sequence of administration of two agents can meaningfully be reversed in order to prove that any enhancement by a second agent truly represents promotion and not syncarcinogenesis.

A wide spectrum of agents has been tested for enhancement of foci in the various models in use (Table III). Most of these studies have used male animals, but there is evidence that for some agents liver promotion may be more effective in females (Deml and Oesterle, 1982). Also, it is noteworthy that phenobarbital, which is a strong

TABLE III

EFFECT OF CHEMICALS STUDIED FOR ENHANCEMENT OF ALTERED FOCI IN RODENT LIVER

Chemical	Species	Effect[a]	References
Acetaminophen	Rat	−	Tsuda *et al.* (1984)
Barbiturates			
Amobarbital	Rat	+	Shinozuka *et al.* (1982)
Barbital	Rat	+	Mori *et al.* (1981)
Barbituric acid	Rat	+	Shinozuka *et al.* (1982)
Pentobarbital	Rat	+	Shinozuka *et al.* (1982)
Phenobarbital	Rat	+	Watanabe and Williams (1978)
Benzodiazepines			
Clorazepate	Rat	−	Mazue *et al.* (1982)
Diazapam	Rat	−	Mazue *et al.* (1982)
Lorazepam	Rat	−	Mazue *et al.* (1982)
Oxazepam	Rat	−	Mazue *et al.* (1982)
Bile acids			
Deoxycholate	Rat	+	Cameron *et al.* (1982)
Lithocholate	Rat	w	Cameron *et al.* (1982)
Butylated hydroxyanisole	Rat	−	Tsuda *et al.* (1984)
Dibromoethane	Rat	+	Milks *et al.* (1982)
Di(2-ethylhexyl)phthalate	Rat	−	DeAngelo and Garrett (1983)
Estrogens			
Estradiol	Rat	−	Yager *et al.* (1984)
Ethinyl estradiol	Rat	+	Yager *et al.* (1984)
Mestranol	Rat	+	Yager *et al.* (1984)
Ethoxyquin	Rat	−	Tsuda *et al.* (1984)
Hexachlorobenzene	Rat	+	Pereira *et al.* (1982a)
Hypolipidemic drugs			
Clofibrate	Rat	±	Numoto *et al.* (1984)
Nafenopin	Rat	−	Numoto *et al.* (1984)
Organochlorine compounds			
Lindane	Rat	+	Pereira *et al.* (1982a)
Chlordane	Mouse	−	Williams and Numoto (1984)
Heptachlor	Mouse	−	Williams and Numoto (1984)
DDT	Mouse	−	Williams and Numoto (1984)
Methapyrilene	Rat	+	Couri *et al.* (1982)
Orotic acid	Rat	+	Columbano *et al.* (1982)
Polychlorinated biphenyls	Rat	+	Pereira *et al.* (1982b)
Saccharin	Rat	−	Tatematsu *et al.* (1983)
Steroid hormones			
Cortisone	Rat	w	Cameron *et al.* (1982)
Dexamethasone	Rat	+	Cameron *et al.* (1982)
Testosterone	Rat	+	Cameron *et al.* (1982)
2,3,7,8-Tetrachlorodibenzo-*p*-dioxin	Rat	+	Pitot *et al.* (1980)
12-*O*-Tetradecanoyl-phorbol-13-acetate	Rat	−	Tatematsu *et al.* (1983)

[a] −, Negative; +, positive; w, weak positive.

promoter of rat liver carcinogenesis, was inactive in the hamster (Stenbäck *et al.,* 1986). In current work, this finding has been confirmed and extended to DDT (Tanaka *et al.,* in preparation).

The enhancement of foci by a nongenotoxic agent when given after, but not before a genotoxic carcinogen demonstrates a promoting action. Nevertheless, many and perhaps all "promoters" can increase the incidence of neoplasms under conditions of chronic exposure (Weisburger and Williams, 1980). In the liver, this effect is probably the result of the promotion of preexisting transformed cells (Williams, 1980), which are manifested by the development of altered foci and neoplasms in untreated animals. Regardless, by the operational definition of carcinogenesis, production of neoplasms establishes a compound as a carcinogen. For this reason, in the classification of carcinogens described above, promoters are designated as a class of epigenetic carcinogens lacking the ability to react with and damage DNA. Therefore, the demonstration of promoting action may be regarded as a means of distinguishing oncogenic agents with this property from genotoxic carcinogens.

VI. Inhibition of Altered Foci as a Means of Identifying Anticarcinogens

Narita *et al.* (1980) reported that administration of phenobarbital together with 3′-methyl-4-(dimethylamino)-azobenzene reduced the number of foci induced by the carcinogen. Maeura *et al.* (1984) showed that butylated hydroxytoluene inhibited *N*-2-fluorenylacetamide induction of foci and, in addition, that the eventual incidence of liver neoplasms was also reduced. Thus, it has been established that inhibition of foci induction is predictive of inhibition of hepatocarcinogenesis.

Up to the present, only a few chemicals given in conjunction with liver carcinogens have been shown to inhibit foci (Table IV). A curious situation is the reports that hypolipidemic agents (Staubli *et al.,* 1984; Perera and Shinozuka, 1984) and acetaminophen (Kurata *et al.,* 1985) given after a carcinogen cause disappearance of foci. In these studies, GGT was used as the marker, and in light of the finding that nafenopin inhibits GGT activity (Numoto *et al.,* 1984; Furukawa *et al.,* 1985), it may be that the foci were made undetectable by the GGT reaction.

TABLE IV

INHIBITION OF ALTERED FOCI IN RODENT LIVER BY CHEMICALS GIVEN IN CONJUNCTION WITH A LIVER CARCINOGEN

Chemical	Carcinogen	Sequence[a]	References
Acetaminophen	*N*-Ethyl-*N*-hydroxy-ethylnitrosamine	FC	Tsuda *et al.* (1984)
	Diethylnitrosamine	FC	Kurata *et al.* (1985)
o-Aminophenol	Diethylnitrosamine	FC	Kurata *et al.* (1985)
m-Aminophenol	Diethylnitrosamine	FC	Kurata *et al.* (1985)
p-Aminophenol	Diethylnitrosamine	FC	Kurata *et al.* (1985)
BR 931	Diethylnitrosamine	FC	Perera and Shinozuka (1984)
	N-2-Fluorenylacetamide	FC	
Butylated hydroxyanisole	*N*-Ethyl-*N*-hydroxy-ethylnitrosamine	FC	Tsuda *et al.* (1984)
	Aflatoxin B_1	WC	Williams *et al.* (1986)
Butylated hydroxytoluene	*N*-2-Fluorenylacetamide	WC	Maeura *et al.* (1984)
	Aflatoxin B_1	WC	Williams *et al.* (1986)
Ethoxyquin	*N*-Ethyl-*N*-hydroxy-ethylnitrosamine	FC	Tsuda *et al.* (1984)
Glucosinolates	Aflatoxin B_1	WC	Godlewski *et al.* (1985)
Nafenopin	Diethylnitrosamine	FC	Staubli *et al.* (1984)
Phenobarbital	3′-Methyl-4-(dimethyl-amino)-azobenzene	WC	Narita *et al.* (1980)

[a]FC, Following carinogen; WC, with carcinogen.

VII. Conclusions

Liver altered foci have been established to be an abnormal population of cells related to hepatocytes that can be produced by liver carcinogens in mice, rats, hamsters, and monkeys. They appear to be precursors of both benign adenomas and carcinomas. In particular, hyperbasophilic foci may be related to carcinomas. Similar lesions have been reported in humans (Hirota *et al.*, 1982) and may be the precursors of hepatocellular carcinomas.

The rapid induction of foci in experimental animals can be used to identify genotoxic carcinogens. Also, the enhancement of foci induced by a genotoxic carcinogen can be used to identify promoters and the inhibition of induction of foci can serve to reveal anticarcinogens.

Acknowledgments

The author thanks his many co-workers, who are evident from the reference list, for their valuable collaboration. Dr. T. Tanaka kindly contributed the photomicrographs for this paper. Mrs. J. Martin and T. Seppell provided dedicated and invaluable services in the preparation of the paper.

References

Abelev, G. I. (1971). *Adv. Cancer Res.* **14,** 295–358.

Astrom, A., DePierre, J. W., and Iriksson, L. (1983). *Carcinogenesis* **4,** 577–581.

Bannasch, P. (1968). *Recaut Cancer Res.* **19,** 1–100.

Barbason, H., and Betz, E. H. (1981). *Br. J. Cancer* **44,** 561–566.

Berenblum, I. (1974). "Carcinogenesis as a Biological Problem," pp. 43–49. North Holland/American Elsevier, Amsterdam.

Boelsterli, U., and Zbinden, G. (1979). "Fine Needle Aspiration Biopsy of the Rat Liver" (G. Zbinden, ed.), pp. 17–31. Pergamon, Oxford.

Bolt, H. M., Laib, R. J., and Stöckle, G. (1979). *Arch. Toxicol.* **43,** 83–84.

Bursch, W., Lauer, B., Timmermann-Trosiener, I., Barthel, G., Schuppler, J., and Schulte-Hermann, R. (1984). *Carcinogenesis* **5,** 453–458.

Butler, W. H., and Newberne, P. M., eds. (1975). "Mouse Hepatic Neoplasia." Elsevier, Amsterdam.

Cameron, R. G., Imaida, K., Tsuda, H., and Ito, I. (1982). *Cancer Res.* **42,** 2426–2428.

Cater, K. C., Gandolfi, A. T., and Sipes, I. G. (1985). *Toxicol. Pathol.* **13,** 3–9.

Columbano, A., Ledda, G. M., Rao, P. M., Rajalakshmi, S., and Sarma, D. S. R. (1982). *Cancer Lett.* **16,** 191–196.

Couri, D., Wilt, S. R., and Milks, M. M. (1982). *Res. Commun. Chem. Pathol. Pharmacol.* **35,** 51–61.

DeAngelo, A. B., and Garrett, C. T. (1983). *Cancer Lett.* **20,** 199–205.

Deml, E., and Oesterle, D. (1982). *Carcinogenesis* **3,** 1449–1453.

Dempo, K., Hisaka, N., Yoshida, Y., Kaneko, A., and Onoe, T. (1975). *Cancer Res.* **35,** 1282–1287.

Doull, J., Bridges, B. A., Kroes, R., Golberg, L., Munro, I. C., Paynter, O. E., Pitot, H. C., Squire, R., and Williams, G. M. (1983). "The Relevance of Mouse Liver Hepatoma to Human Carcinogenic Risk." Nutrition Foundation, Washington, D.C.

Emmelot, P., and Scherer, E. (1980). *Biochim. Biophys. Acta* **605,** 247–304.

Farber, E. (1956). *Cancer Res.* **7,** 142–155.

Farber, E. (1973). *lethods Cancer Res.* **7,** 345–375.

Farber, E. (1979). "Toxic Injury of the Liver" (E. Farber and M. M. Fisher, eds.), pp. 445–467. Dekker, New York.

Farber, E., Parker, S., and Gruenstein, M. (1979). *Cancer Res.* **36,** 3879.

Fiala, S., Mohindru, A., and Kettering, W. G. (1976). *J. Natl. Cancer Inst.* **57,** 591–598.

Firminger, H. I. (1955). *J. Natl. Cancer Inst.* **15,** 1427–1442.

Friedrich-Freksa, S. H., Gossner, W., and Borner, P. (1969). *Z. Krebsforsch.* **72,** 226–239.

Furukawa, K., Maeura, Y., Furukawa, N. T., and Williams, G. M. (1984). *Chem. Biol. Interact.* **48,** 43–58.

Furukawa, K., Numoto, S., Furuya, K., Furukawa, N., and Williams, G. M. (1985). *Cancer Res.* **45,** 5011–5019.

Furuya, K., and Williams, G. M. (1984). *Toxicol. Appl. Pharmacol.* **74,** 63–69.

Furuya, K., Maeura, Y., and Williams, G. M. (1984). *Toxicol. Pathol.* **12,** 136–142.

Godlewski, C. E., Boyd, J. N., Sherman, W. K., Anderson, J. L., and Stoewsand, G. S. (1985). *Cancer Lett.* **28,** 151–157.

Gössner, V. W., and Friedrich-Freksa, H. (1964). *Z. Naturforsch.* **19b,** 862–863.

Grisham, J. W., and Hartroft, W. S. (1961). *Lab. Invest.* **10,** 317–332.

Grisham, J. W., and Porta, E. A. (1964). *Exp. Mol. Pathol.* **3,** 242–261.

Guillouzo, A., Weber, A., Le Provost, E., Rissel, M., and Schapira, F. (1981). *J. Cell Sci.* **49,** 249–260.

Haddow, A. (1938). *Acta Uni. Int. Cancrum* **3,** 342–352.

Harada, M., Okabe, K., Shibata, K., Masuda, H., Miyata, K., and Enomoto, M. (1976). *Acta Histochem.* **9,** 168–179.

Herren, S. L., Pereira, M. A., Britt, A. L., and Khoury, M. K. (1982). *Toxicol. Lett.* **12,** 143–150.

Hirota, N., and Williams, G. M. (1979a). *J. Natl. Cancer Inst.* **63,** 1257–1265.

Hirota, N., and Williams, G. M. (1979b). *Am. J. Pathol.* **95,** 317–324.

Hirota, N., and Williams, G. M. (1982). *Cancer Res.* **42,** 2298–2309.

Hirota, N., Hamazaki, M., and Williams, G. M. (1982). *Hepatogastroenterology* **29,** 49–51.

Hunt, J. M., and Laishes, B. A. (1982). "Toxicology of the Liver" (G. Plaa and W. R. Hewitt eds.), pp. 291–309. Raven, New York.

Inaoka, Y. (1967). *Gann* **58,** 355–366.

Ishikawa, T., Takayama, S., Kitagawa, T., Kawachi, T., and Sugimura, T. (1979). *J. Cancer Res. Clin. Oncol.* **95,** 221–224.

Jones, Jr., D. E., Evces, S., and Lindahl, R. (1984). *Carcinogenesis* **5,** 1679–1687.

Judah, D. J., Legg, R. F., and Neal, G. E. (1977). *Nature (London)* **265,** 343–345.

Kalengayi, M. M. R., Rochi, G., and Desmet, V. J. (1975). *J. Natl. Cancer Inst.* **55,** 579–588.

Katayama, S., Ohmori, T., Maeura, Y., Croci, T., and Williams, G. M. (1984). *J. Natl. Cancer Inst.* **73,** 141–149.

Kitagawa, T. (1971). *Gann* **62,** 207–216.

Kitagawa, T., and Sugano, H. (1978). *Gann* **69,** 679–687.

Kitagawa, T., Yokochi, T., and Sugano, H. (1972). *Int. J. Cancer* **10,** 368–381.

Kitahara, A., Satoh, K., and Sato, J. (1983). *Biochem. Biophys. Res. Commun.* **112,** 20–28.

Kitahara, A., Satoh, K., Nishimura, K., Ishikawa, T., Ruike, K., Sata, K., Tsuda, H., and Ito, N. (1984). *Cancer Res.* **44,** 2698–2703.

Kroes, R., Williams, G. M., and Weisburger, J. H. (1972). *Cancer Res.* **32,** 1526–1532.

Kroes, R., Williams, G. M., and Weisburger, J. H. (1973). *Cancer Res.* **33,** 613–617.

Kuchlbauer, J., Romen, W., and Neumann, H. G. (1985). *Carcinogenesis* **6,** 1337–1342.

Kuhlmann, W. D. (1978). *Int. J. Cancer* **21,** 368–380.

Kuhlmann, W. D., Krischan, R., Kunz, W., Guenther, T. M., and Oesch, F. (1981). *Biochem. Biophys. Res. Commun.* **98,** 417–423.

Kurata, Y., Tsuda, H., Tamamo, S., and Ito, N. (1985). *Cancer Lett.* **28,** 19–25.

Laib, R. J., Stöckle, G., Bolt, H. M., and Kunz, W. (1979). *J. Cancer Res. Clin. Oncol.* **94,** 139–147.

Leonard, T. B., Dent, J. G., Graichen, M. E., Lyght, O., and Popp, J. A. (1982). *Carcinogenesis* **3,** 851–856.

Lipsky, M. M., Hinton, D. E., Goldblatt, P. J., Klaunig, J. E., and Trump, B. F. (1979). *Pathol. Res. Pract.* **164,** 178–185.

Lipsky, M. M., Hinton, D. E., Klaunig, J. E., Goldblatt, P. J., and Trump, B. F. (1980). *Carcinogenesis* **1,** 151–156.

Lopez, M., and Mazzanti, L. (1955). *J. Pathol. Bacteriol.* **69,** 243–250.

Maeura, Y., and Williams, G. M. (1984). *Food Chem. Toxicol.* **22,** 191–198.

Maeura, Y., Weisburger, J. H., and Williams, G. M. (1984). *Cancer Res.* **44,** 1604–1610.

Malvaldi, G. (1981). *Eur. J. Cancer* **17,** 481–483.

Mazue, G., Remandet, B., Gouy, D., Berthe, J., Roncucci, R., and Williams, G. M. (1982). *Arch. Int. Pharm. Ther.* **257,** 59–65.

Milks, M. M., Wilt, S. R., Ali, I., Pereira, M. A., and Couri, D. (1982). *Arch. Toxicol.* **51,** 27–35.

Moore, M. R., Drinkwater, N. R., Miller, E. C., Miller, J. A., and Pitot, H. C. (1981). *Cancer Res.* **41,** 1585–1593.

Mori, M. A., Mayer, D., and Bannasch, P. (1982). *Carcinogenesis* **3,** 1429–1436.

Mori, H., Tanaka, T., Nishikawa, A., Takahashi, M., and Williams, G. M. (1981). *Gann* **72,** 798–801.

Mori, H., Tanaka, T., Sugie, S., Takahashi, M., and Williams, G. M. (1982a). *J. Natl. Cancer Inst. 69,* 1277–1282.

Mori, H., Mu, B., and Williams, G. M. (1982b). *Exp. Mol. Pathol.* **37,** 101–110.

Mori, H., Furuya, K., and Williams, G. M. (1983). *J. Natl. Cancer Inst.* **71,** 849–854.

Mori, H., Sugie, S., Ohbayashi, F., Shima, H., Yoahimi, N., Takahashi, M., and Williams, G. M. (1985a). *Carcinogenesis* **6,** 1087–1090.

Mori, H., Kuniyasu, T., Sugie, S., Shima, H., and Takahashi, M. (1985b). *Carcinogenesis* **6,** 1529–1531.

Narita, T., Watanabe, R., and Kitagawa, T. (1980). *Gann* **71,** 755–758.

Newberne, P. M., and Wogan, G. N. (1968). *Cancer Res.* **28,** 770–781.

Nigam, S. K., Babu, K. A., Bhatt, D. K. *et al.* (1981). *Indian J. Med. Res.* **74,** 289–296.

Numoto, S., Furukawa, K., Furuya, K., and Williams, G. M. (1984). *Carcinogenesis* **5,** 1603–1611.

Numoto, S., Tanaka, T., and Williams, G. M. (1985a). *Toxicol. Pathol.* **13,** 325–334.

Numoto, S., Mori, H., Furuya, K., Levine, W. G., and Williams, G. M. (1985b). *Toxicol. Appl. Pharmacol.* **77,** 76–85.

Ogawa, K., Solt, D. B., and Farber, E. (1980). *Cancer Res.* **40,** 725–732.

Ogawa, K., Onoi, T., and Tabeuchi, J. (1981). *J. Natl. Cancer Inst.* **67,** 407–412.

Ohmori, T., Rice, J. M., and Williams, G. M. (1981). *Histochem. J.* **13,** 85–99.

Okita, K., Noda, K., Fukomoto, Y., and Takemato, T. (1976). *Gann* **67,** 899–902.

Peraino, C., Staffeldt, E. F., and Ludeman, V. A. (1981). *Carcinogenesis* **2,** 463–465.

Peraino, C., Staffeldt, E. F., Carnes, B. A., Ludeman, V. A., Blomquist, J. A., and Vesselinovitch, S. D. (1984). *Cancer Res.* **44,** 3340–3347.

Pereira, M. A. (1982). *J. Am. Coll. Toxicol.* **1,** 101–118.

Pereira, M. A., and Stoner, G. D. (1985). *Fundam. Appl. Toxicol.* **5,** 688–699.

Perera, M. I. R., and Shinozuka, H. (1984). *Carcinogenesis* **5,** 1193–1198.

Pereira, M. A., Herren, S. L., Britt, A. L., and Khoury, M. M. (1982a). *Cancer Lett.* **15,** 95–101.

Pereira, M. A., Herren, S. L., Britt, A. L., and Khoury, M. M. (1982b). *Cancer Lett.* **15,** 185–190.

Pitot, H. C., and Sirica, A. E. (1980). *Biochim. Biophys. Acta* **604,** 191–215.

Pitot, H. C., Barsness, L., Goldsworthy, T., and Kitagawa, T. (1978). *Nature (London)* **271,** 456–458.

Pitot, H. C., Goldsworthy, T., Campbell, H. A., and Poland, A. (1980). *Cancer Res.* **40,** 3616–3620.

Pugh, T. D., and Goldfarb, S. (1978). *Cancer Res.* **38,** 4450–4457.

Rabes, H. M., and Szymkowiak, R. (1979). *Cancer Res.* **39,** 1298–1304.

Rabes, H., Scholze, P., and Jantsch, B. (1972). *Cancer Res.* **32,** 2577–2586.

Rabes, H. M., Bucher, T., Hartmann, A., Linke, I., and Dunnwold, M. (1982). *Cancer Res.* **42,** 3220–3227.

Reilly, C. A., Jr., Peraino, C., Haugen, D. A., Mahlum, D. D., and Springer, D. L. (1985). *Cancer Lett.* **28,** 121–125.

Remandet, B., Gouy, D., Berthe, J., Mazue, G., and Williams, G. M. (1984). *Fundam. Appl. Toxicol.* **4,** 152–163.

Reuber, M. D. (1965). *J. Natl. Cancer Inst.* **34,** 697–724.

Ruebner, B. H., Michas, C., Kanayama, R., and Bannasch, P. (1976). *J. Natl. Cancer Inst.* **53,** 1261–1267.

Rubin, E. (1964). *Exp. Mol. Pathol.* **3,** 279–286.

Scherer, E., Hoffmann, M., Emmelot, P., and Friedrich-Freksa, M. (1972). *J. Natl. Cancer Inst.* **49,** 93–106.

Schulte-Hermann, R., Ohde, G., Schuppler, J., and Timmermann-Trosiener, I. (1981). *Cancer Res.* **41,** 2556–2562.

Schwarz, M., Bannasch, P., and Kunz, W. (1983). *Cancer Lett.* **21,** 17–21.

Sell, S. (1978). *Cancer Res.* **38,** 3107–3113.

Sell, S., Leffert, H. L., Shinozuka, H., Lombardi, B., and Gochman, N. (1981). *Gann* **72,** 479–487.

Shinozuka, H., Lombardi, B., Sell, S., and Iammarino, R. M. (1978). *Cancer Res.* **38,** 1092–1098.

Shinozuka, H., Sells, M. A., Katyal, S. L., Sells, S., and Lombardi, B. (1979) *Cancer Res.* **39,** 2512–2521.

Shinozuka, H., Lombardi, B., and Abanobi, S. E. (1982). *Carcinogenesis* **3,** 1017–1020.

Shirai, T., Hosodo, K., Hirose, K., Hirose, M., and Ito, N. (1985). *Cancer Lett.* **28,** 127–133.

Squire, R. A., and Levitt, M. H. (1975). *Cancer Res.* **35,** 3214–3233.

Staubli, W., Bentley, P., Bieri, F., Frehlich, E., and Waechter, F. (1984). *Carcinogenesis* **5,** 41–46.

Stenbäck, F., Mori, H., Furuya, K., and Williams, G. M. (1986). *J. Natl. Cancer Inst.* **76,** 327–333.

Stewart, H. L., Williams, G. M., Keysser, C. H., Lombard, L. S., and Montali R. J. (1980). *J. Natl. Cancer Inst.* **64,** 177–207.

Takahashi, S., Lombardi, B., and Shinozuka, H. (1982). *Int. J. Cancer* **29,** 445–450.
Tatematsu, M., Shirai, T., Tsuda, H., Miyata, Y., Shinohara, Y., and Ito, N. (1977). *Gann* **68,** 499–507.
Tatematsu, M., Takano, T., Hasegawa, R., Imaida, K., Nakanowatari, J., and Ito, N. (1980). *Gann* **71,** 843–855.
Tatematsu, M., Hasegawa, R., Imaida, K., Tsuda, H., and Ito, N. (1983). *Carcinogenesis* **4,** 381–386.
Tchipysheva, T. A., Guelstein, V. I., and Bannikov, G. A. (1977). *Int. J. Cancer* **20,** 388–393.
Teebor, G. W., and Becker, F. F. (1971). *Cancer Res.* **31,** 1–3.
Telang, S., Tong, C., and Williams, G. M. (1982). *Carcinogenesis* **3,** 1175–1178.
Timme, A. H. (1978). *J. Natl. Cancer Inst.* **61,** 407–408.
Tsuda, H., Lee, G., and Farber, E. (1980). *Cancer Res.* **40,** 1157–1164.
Tsuda, H., Sakata, T., Masui, T., Imaida, K., and Ito, N. (1984). *Carcinogenesis* **5,** 525–531.
Vasiliev, J. M., and Guelstein, V. I. (1963). *J. Natl. Cancer Inst.* **31,** 1123–1143.
Wanson, J. C., de Ridder, L., and Mosselmans, R. (1981). *Cancer Res.* **41,** 5162–5175.
Ward, J. M. (1981). *Virchows Arch. A. Pathol. Anat.* **390,** 339–345.
Watabe, H. (1971). *Cancer Res.* **31,** 1192–1194.
Watanabe, K., and Williams, G. M. (1978). *J. Natl. Cancer Inst.* **61,** 1311–1314.
Weisburger, J. H., and Williams, G. M. (1980). "Toxicology. The Basic Science of Poisons" (J. Doull, C. D. Klaasen, and M. O. Amdur, eds.), 2nd Ed., pp. 84–138. Macmillan, New York.
Weisburger, J. H., and Williams, G. M. (1981). *Science* **214,** 401–407.
Williams, G. M. (1976). *Cancer Res.* **36,** 2540–2543.
Williams, G. M. (1980). *Biochim. Biophys, Acta* **605,** 167–189.
Williams, G. M. (1982). *Toxicol. Pathol.* **10,** 3–10.
Williams, G. M. (1984). *Fundam. Appl. Toxicol.* **4,** 325–344.
Williams, G. M., and Furuya, K. (1984). *Carcinogenesis* **5,** 171–174.
Williams, G. M. and Numoto, S. (1984). *Carcinogenesis* **5,** 1689–1696.
Williams, G. M., and Watanabe, K. (1978). *J. Natl. Cancer Inst.* **61,** 113–121.
Williams, G. M., and Weisburger, J. H. (1981). *Annu. Rev. Pharmacol. Toxicol.* **21,** 393–416.
Williams, G. M., and Yamamoto, R. S. (1972). *J. Natl. Cancer Inst.* **49,** 685–692.
Williams, G. M., Klaiber, M., Parker, S. E., and Farber, E. (1976). *J. Natl. Cancer Inst.* **57,** 157–165.
Williams, G. M., Klaiber, M., and Farber E. (1977). *Am. J. Pathol.* **89,** 379–388.
Williams, G. M., Hirota, N., and Rice, J. (1979). *Am. J. Pathol.* **94,** 65–74.
Williams, G. M, Ohmori, T., and Watanabe, K. (1980). *Am. J. Pathol.* **99,** 1–12.
Williams, G. M., Katayama, S., and Ohmori, T. (1981). *Carcinogenesis* **2,** 1111–1117.
Williams, G. M., Tanaka, T., and Maeura, Y. (1986). *Carcinogenesis* **7,** 1043–1050.
Yager, J. D., Campbell, H. A., Longnecker, D. S., Roebuck, B. D., and Benoit, M. C. (1984). *Cancer Res.* **44,** 3862–3869.

ADVANCES IN VETERINARY SCIENCE AND COMPARATIVE MEDICINE, VOL. 31

Liver Tumors in Rodents: Extrapolation to Man

FRANCIS J. C. ROE

19 Marryat Road, Wimbledon Common, London SW19 5BB, England

I. Introduction

Man is not the species of choice for studies in the field of experimental pathology. He's too big. He costs too much to feed. He is expensive to house and maintain. And he seems bent on actively defying any attempt to carry out a controlled experiment on him as a member of his species. However, the greatest drawback to the use of man as an experimental model is that, although men kill other men freely for political purposes, humans as a species have evolved a thought process known as "ethics" which proscribes interim sacrifice at planned time points in long-term observational studies. Consequently, it is very difficult to trace the origins and pathogenesis of any eventually neoplastic lesion in man and equally difficult to chart the occurrence, persistence, progression, or regression of putatively precancerous lesions.

In the light of these serious limitations, had the second part of the title of this chapter had been "extrapolation *from* man," I would have had to say that man is an extremely inappropriate model for the prediction of liver tumor risk in rats and mice. In fact, there are only a few examples of agents (e.g., steroids, vinyl chloride) which give rise to liver tumors of similar kinds in rodents and humans. Otherwise there is seemingly little overlap between the spectrum of factors which contribute importantly to the causation of liver neoplasia in man and that of factors which do so in rodents. Moreover, whereas liver neoplasia is a rare disease in westernized man, it is relatively common in rodents generally, and actually reaches an incidence of 100% "spontaneously" in some strains of mice.

In this chapter, I propose to start by distinguishing between various types of hepatic neoplasia. Next I will discuss the factors known to be associated with increased risk of liver neoplasia as a human disease, and the extent to which it is known that the same factors have a similar effect in laboratory animals. Finally, against this background, I will consider situations where there are data indicating that a substance possesses hepatocarcinogenic activity for laboratory rodents, but where there are no comparable data for humans.

II. Different Kinds of Liver Tumors

The liver consists mainly of five kinds of cells: (1) parenchymal (also called liver cell), (2) bile duct, (3) blood vessel, (4) reticuloendothelial (called Kupffer cell), and (5) connective tissue.

Each of these cell types may be the origin of benign or malignant tumors. The criteria for distinguishing between benign and malignant neoplasia are considered below. Hepatocellular adenomas (benign) and hepatocellular carcinomas (malignant) arise in parenchymal cells; cholangiomas (benign) and cholangiocarcinomas (malignant) arise in bile duct cells; angiomas or hemangiomas (benign) and angiosarcomas or hemangioendotheliomas (malignant) arise from blood vessel cells; Kupffer cell sarcomas (malignant) arise in reticuloendothelial cells, and sarcomas (malignant) arise in connective tissue cells.

In this chapter we are mainly concerned with tumors arising from parenchymal cells, bile duct cells, and blood vessel cells.

III. Etiological Factors for Hepatic Neoplasia in Man and the Availability of Animal Models

A. Hepatitis B Virus

Although primary liver cancer is relatively rare in Europe and North America, it occurs commonly in certain parts of Asia and Africa. In the areas of high incidence there is also a high incidence of viral hepatitis B infection. There is good evidence that chronic carriers of the hepatitis B virus are prone to develop macronodular cirrhosis and that this tends to progress to hepatocellular carcinoma. The detection of the hepatitis B virus genome both in the DNA of liver cells of carriers and in the DNA of hepatocellular carcinomas (Shafritz and Kew, 1981; Prince, 1981) provides strong evidence of the involvement of the virus in the etiology of the neoplasia. If the virus is vertically transmitted from a mother who is a chronic carrier to her child, then the risk of the child developing a hepatocellular carcinoma is especially high. Furthermore, if the father is negative for surface antibodies to the virus (indicating that he is immunologically defective), then the risk of the child developing a liver cancer is even higher (Larouze *et al.,* 1976).

There is no known parallel for this form of viral hepatocarcinogenesis in rats or mice. However, a form of viral hepatocarcinogenesis in the woodchuck may be a good model. In this species, the introduction of a virus closely resembling the hepatitis B virus leads to the development of chronic viral hepatitis which progresses to macronodular cirrhosis and eventually to hepatocellular carcinoma (Summers, 1981; Johnson and Williams, 1981).

B. Steroids

The occurrence of liver cell tumors, mostly benign and amenable to surgical excision, but occasionally fatal because of intraperitoneal hemorrhage or inoperable malignancy, is well documented for women taking various forms of contraceptive pills (Baum *et al.,* 1973; Neuberger *et al.,* 1980). Similar hepatic neoplasms have been reported in humans exposed to androgens such as oxymethalone and methyltestosterone (Johnson *et al.,* 1972; Farrell *et al.,* 1975; Sweeney and Evans, 1976).

In mice, several contraceptive pill formulations have been found to enhance the incidence of liver cell tumors (Committee on Safety of Medicines, 1972). In most strains or mice, liver tumors arise spontaneously more frequently in males than in females. Castration and the administration of estrogens reduces liver tumor incidence in males while ovariectomy and the administration of androgens increases liver tumor incidence in females (Agnew and Gardner, 1952; Andervont, 1950).

C. Aflatoxin B_1 and Other Aflatoxins

Aflatoxin B_1 and related aflatoxins derived from the mold *Aspergillus flavus* are potent hepatotoxins for many different species (Lancaster *et al.,* 1961; Kraybill and Shimkin, 1964). Even at a level of only 1 μg/kg diet aflatoxin B_1 has been reported to give rise to liver tumors in the rat (Wogan *et al.,* 1974). Aflatoxin B_1 has also been found to cause liver tumors in the rainbow trout (Sinnhuber *et al.,*

1968), in salmon (Wales and Sinnhuber, 1972), and in a few primates (Adamson *et al.*, 1973; Reddy and Svoboda, 1975). Against this background of response in various species, it is, a priori, to be expected that aflatoxin B_1 is a liver carcinogen for man. However, the evidence that this is so is fundamentally no more than circumstantial. Thus, although high levels of aflatoxin have been found in food in geographical areas where liver cancer in humans is common (Linsell, 1978), there is no compelling supportive evidence, as there is in the case of the hepatitis B virus, that the association is causal.

Curiously, although it is easy to produce liver tumors in rats by administering aflatoxins to them by the oral route, mice are resistant to liver tumor induction in this way. Wogan (1969) failed to produce liver tumors either in random-bred or inbred mouse strains by feeding aflatoxin B_1 at a level of 1 mg/kg in the diet. However, Vesselinovitch *et al.* (1972) produced liver tumors in 80% of (C57BL × C3H)F_1 hybrid mice by administering aflatoxin B_1 by the intraperitoneal route during the first 7 days of life.

D. Alcoholic Cirrhosis

An obsession with sin and its consequences has long had the effect of making the theory that cirrhosis due to an excessive intake of alcohol predisposes to primary liver cancer appealing to puritans. Nevertheless, the evidence that this is a common sequence of events is not robust. If all forms of cirrhosis predispose equally to cancer, one might expect there to be a similar relationship between the incidences of cirrhosis and liver cancer in geographically different areas. But this is not so. In certain areas of South Africa, non-Caucasians who develop one or other form of cirrhosis have a 40–50% risk of developing a liver cancer (Thompson, 1961), whereas the comparable figure for Chicago in the United States is only 5% (Stuart, 1965).

There are, in fact, several different varieties of cirrhosis. The form most associated with increased liver cancer risk is the *postnecrotic* or *macronodular* type, whereas the type most commonly associated with alcoholism is the *hobnail* or *finely nodular* type, sometimes referred to as nutritional cirrhosis (Lee, 1966).

Historically, confusion has arisen because alcoholic beverages, particularly when prepared by primitive methods from diseased crops in hot and humid climates, are apt to be contaminated with true carcinogens (e.g., mold toxins, nitrosamines).

Overall, it seems that the risk of liver cancer development in persons who develop nutritional cirrhosis because of an excessive intake of alcohol per se is not very high, unless these persons are also chronic carriers of hepatitis B virus and/or are additionally exposed to some liver toxin, such as aflatoxin. The variation in distributions of cirrhosis and primary liver cancer between the different social classes in England and Wales (see below) are consistent with this conclusion. On the other hand, according to Arrigoni *et al.* (1985), in Italy, hepatocellular carcinoma occurs as commonly in patients with alcoholic cirrhosis who are not infected with hepatitis B virus as in those that are.

In view of the fact that the association between exposure to alcohol and increased liver cancer risk is no more than weak in man, it is not perhaps surprising that cirrhosis and liver tumors are most definitely not responses that are seen in laboratory animals as a consequence of exposure to ethyl alcohol.

Numerous investigators have exposed laboratory animals to high daily doses of ethanol over long periods with very little evidence of adverse effect as far as the liver is concerned. Thus, Ketcham *et al.* (1963) exposed CDBA/$2F_1$ female mice for up to 15 months to 20% (v/v) ethanol instead of drinking water. This treatment had no effect on longevity, primary tumor incidence at any site, or the growth or spread of tumor implants. Moderate fatty infiltration of liver parenchymal cells was seen in the livers of animals killed after 1 year's treatment, but this change partly regressed during a subsequent alcohol-free period. Cirrhosis was not seen. Kuratsune *et al.* (1971) saw no liver tumors among 108 male and 42 female CF_1 strain mice provided intermittently with 43% aqueous solution of ethanol instead of drinking water and observed for up to 34 months. The same investigators also saw no liver tumors in 100 male ddN strain mice given a 19.5% aqueous solution of ethanol intermittently instead of drinking water and observed for up to 22 months.

Schmähl (1976) maintained Sprague–Dawley rats on 30 ml/kg 25% aqueous ethanol in drinking water on 5 days per week for up to 780 days without producing any evidence of hepatotoxic activity or any liver tumors. Earlier, Gibel (1967) exposed 40 Sprague–Dawley rats to 0.5 ml 30% (w/v) ethanol once daily for up to 20 months. Apart from slight liver changes in 10% of the animals after 6 months of treatment, no adverse effects on the liver were encountered.

Herrold (1969) gave 0.5 ml 50% ethanol twice weekly by mouth to five male and five female hamsters for a period of 10–11 months. She then followed the animals for life (average 21 months of age) but observed no adverse effects on the liver.

Hollander and Higginson (1971) gave 10% aqueous ethanol instead of drinking water to 19 male and 33 female mastomys for 2 months and then increased the concentration to 20% for the remainder of their life span (up to 30 months). The incidence of malignant carcinoid tumors of the stomach, to which this species is prone, was not adversely affected by the exposure to ethanol and none of the treated animals developed primary tumors of the liver.

In reviewing the weakness of the association between alcohol consumption and liver cancer risk in man and the lack of any evidence for such an association in laboratory animals, I should make it clear that my comments do not necessarily apply to the more substantial evidence for a causal association between alcohol consumption and risk of cancer development at other sites (e.g., head and neck) in man (Maclure and MacMahon, 1980; Tuyns, 1979). However, in relation to these forms of cancer, also, the question of whether the association between these cancers and alcohol consumption is indicative of carcinogenesis by alcohol *per se,* or by contamination of alcoholic beverages by carcinogens, or by some other mechanism, needs to be seriously addressed.

E. Vinyl Chloride

Heavy exposure to vinyl chloride is associated with an increased risk of angiosarcoma of the liver in humans, rats, and mice (Creech and Johnson, 1974; Maltoni, 1977). Vinyl chloride is a genotoxic agent, and the assumption is that the liver tumors are a direct consequence of this activity.

F. Thorium Dioxide

Thorotrast (thorium-232 dioxide) was at one time used as a radiographic contrast medium to outline body cavities such as the renal pelvis or for the visualization of blood vessels. Once introduced into the tissues, thorium is taken up by reticuloendothelial cells throughout the body, including the Kupffer cells of the liver. These cells thereafter become sources of radiation with which they bombard surrounding cells and thereby increase the risk of their mutation to cancerous cells. Thus, patients who have received thorotrast are at increased risk for developing various kinds of primary liver cancer. Boyd *et al.* (1968) reported 3 cases of cholangiocarcinoma arising in intrahepatic bile ducts and 1 case of hepatic hemangioendothelioma among 109 patients who survived for at least 1 year after receiving thorotrast. Numerous other anecdotal cases of primary liver cancer arising following thorotrast administration are to be found in the literature (e.g., MacMahon *et al.*, 1947; Nettleship and Fink, 1961; Stemmermann, 1960).

Doubtless the liver would be among the sites for the development of neoplasms in rats and mice were a properly designed study which mimicked human exposure to thorotrast undertaken. Unfortunately, no such study has been reported in the literature in either of these species. On the other hand, Swarm *et al.* (1962) reported hepatic hemangioendotheliomas in two of three female rabbits given intravenous thorotrast.

IV. Mortality from Primary Liver Cancer in England and Wales

In 1984 there were 479 deaths in males and 231 deaths in females from primary cancer of the liver [International Classification of Diseases, ninth revision (ICD, No. 155.0)]. Corresponding figures in 1974 (311 deaths in males, 196 in females) and in 1964 (265 deaths in males, 164 in females) showed that there seems to have been some increase in both sexes. There were also a further 148 deaths in each sex from cancer of intrahepatic bile ducts in 1984 (ICD 155.1), a figure markedly higher than the 21 male and 34 female cases recorded in 1974. Earlier figures for cancer of this site are not available. In 1984 there were also 86 deaths in males and 87 deaths in females where the cancer was not specified as primary or secondary (ICD 155.2). According to Case (1956), the age-standardized mortality from cancers of the liver and gallbladder in England and Wales fell in both men and women belonging to successive quinary–quinquennial cohorts with birth dates centered on 1871, 1881, 1891, and 1901. The contrast with the more recent trends may reflect the changing pattern of alcohol consumption over this century with a sharp decline from the high levels at the beginning of the century, followed by a marked rise over the last two or three decades.

In addition to deaths diagnosed as primary liver, there were also in 1984 a further 1210 deaths in males and 1070 in females classified as of chronic liver disease of cirrhosis (ICD 571). These also showed an increase over the corresponding figures for 1974 (901 deaths in males and 853 in females) and in 1964 (657 deaths in males and 652 in females). Of the 1984 deaths, the major contributions were from alcoholic cirrhosis of the liver (ICD 571.2, 435 male and 242 female deaths), cirrhosis with no mention of liver (ICD 571.5, 517 male and and 409 female deaths), alcoholic liver damage unspecified (ICD 571.3, 101 male and 70 female deaths), and biliary cirrhosis (ICD 571.6, 28 male and 182 female deaths), but it is not possible to study trends in these due to changes in the ICD classifications used in compiling the mortality data. Unfortunately, the death certificate data from which these totals were compiled are not detailed or reliable enough to throw useful light on the relationship between liver cancer and cirrhosis. In any event, it is clear that the liver is the primary site of only a very small proportion of fatal neoplasms in humans in England and Wales: deaths in ICD 155.0, 155.1, and 155.2 combined formed only 1179 of a total of 140,101, about 0.8%.

According to the Registrar General's decennial supplement on Occupational Mortality in England and Wales for 1970–1972 (Registrar General, 1978) for men aged 15–64, there is little difference between social classes I–III in risk of death from primary liver cancer, but for men in semiskilled occupations (social class IV), the standardized mortality ratio (SMR) is slightly increased, while for men in unskilled occupations (social class V), the 61 deaths that were observed were over 50% higher than the 39 expected for men as a whole. By comparison, the SMR for men in the same age group for cirrhosis of the liver is highest in social class II (almost 150), second highest in social class V (120), and lowest in social classes IIIB and IV. Obviously, there is a very poor relationship between the distribution of deaths for, on the one hand, liver cancer and, on the other hand, cirrhosis between the social classes. These data are consistent with the conclusion reached earlier that the association between alcoholic cirrhosis and risk of developing primary liver cancer is relatively weak.

V. Factors Other Than Test Chemicals Which Influence the Risk of Hepatic Neoplasia in Laboratory Rodents

Tumors originating in the various kinds of liver cells are commonly found in laboratory rats and mice which have not been deliberately exposed to any potentially carcinogenic agent. The causation of these apparently "spontaneously arising" tumors in rats and mice is no less a mystery than the causation of many kinds of cancer in man. However, a number of factors which influence the incidence of these "spontaneous" tumors have been identified, and it is important to consider and discuss these factors for two reasons. First, it is well recognized that in laboratory animals it is easier to increase the incidence of tumors of kinds that occur "spontaneously" in high incidence than that of tumors that occur "spontaneously" only in low incidence. This suggests that the primary and most important causal factor of high-incidence tumors may already be present in the test system. This being so, a variety of additional relatively weak stimuli may, perhaps nonspecifically, promote the "germination" of tumors, the seeds of which are already present in the test system. Second, if it is known that certain nonspecific factors (e.g., calorie intake, fat intake, sex hormone status; see below) influence liver tumor risk, then one must expect that test materials which bring about changes in the status of animals with respect to these factors will also, indirectly, affect liver tumor risk.

Before we consider nonspecific environmental factors, however, we need briefly to mention genetic influences including male–female differences in incidence.

A. Genetic Constitution

Different inbred strains of mice have remarkably different incidences of "spontaneous" liver tumors, with some strains (e.g., C3H) exhibiting a lifetime expectation of developing one or more parenchymal cell tumors of up to 100% in both sexes and other strains exhibiting an almost zero lifetime incidence (Andervont, 1950; Grasso and Hardy, 1975). Some of the exceptionally high liver tumor-susceptible strains were, in fact, purposely developed by selective inbreeding. However, even wild house mice bred in captivity are not free from liver tumor risk. Andervont and Dunn (1962) reported a 3.5% incidence of hepatomas in female house mice living to a mean age of 30 months and a 9% incidence of males living to a mean of 23 months. These incidences are much higher than for humans living in Europe or North America.

Strain differences in spontaneous liver tumor risk are also evident in rats but are less well documented. In general, the very high incidences of "spontaneous" liver cell tumors found in some strains of mice are not encountered in rats, although I have seen incidences as high as 16% in untreated male and 29% in untreated female rats of a Wistar strain.

B. Sex

In most strains of mice, males are more susceptible to the spontaneous development of liver tumors than females. Furthermore, manipulation of hormonal status (e.g., by ovariectomy and/or androgen administration in females and by orchidectomy and/or estrogen administration in males) affects the risk of spontaneous liver tumor development in the direction of a higher risk being associated with increase in masculinity (Agnew and Gardner, 1952).

In the case of most strains of rats, the sexes are seemingly more or less equal in their chances of developing liver cell tumors "spontaneously," with females tending to be slightly more at risk (e.g., Goodman *et al.,* 1979).

C. Dietary Intake: Effects of Overnutrition and Fat Intake in Mice

It has long been known from the classical studies of Tannenbaum and Silverstone that the risk of development of many kinds of neoplasms in mice is influenced by the composition of the diet and by caloric intake. Among the kinds of neoplasms influenced by dietary intake and the composition of the diet (e.g., levels of casein) is the liver cell tumor of mice. Tannenbaum (1940, 1947) suggested that diet restriction may act to reduce liver tumor incidence in mice via a hormonal mechanism. This theory was supported by the observation of Heston (1963) that the occurrence of hepatomas in the highly susceptible (C3H × YBR)F_1 male mouse was completely inhibited by hypophysectomy and also by the finding in the same strain of mice by Rowlatt *et al.* (1973) that diet restriction without endocrine ablation inhibited liver tumor risk.

Diets containing 18% or 45% casein have been found to lead to higher incidences of liver cell tumors in mice of either sex than a diet containing only 9% casein (Tannenbaum and Silverstone, 1949). The effect was observed irrespective of whether the animals were fed *ad libitum* or isocalorically.

The concentration of fat in the diet may have an even more dramatic effect on the "spontaneous" incidence of liver cell tumors in mice (Sokoloff *et al.,* 1960). In one study by Gellatly (1975), when the percentage of ground nut oil incorporated into a semisynthetic diet fed to C57BL mice was increased from 5% to 10%, survival to 80 weeks decreased but the percentage of survivors exhibiting benign or malignant liver cell tumors increased dramatically, particularly in females (see Table I).

More recently, Conybeare (1980), in a large study on random-bred Swiss mice, compared the effects of *ad libitum* feeding of two standard laboratory diets with those of restricting animals to only 75% of the food consumed by the *ad libitum*-fed animals. He recorded consistent beneficial effects of diet restriction on both survival and percentage of survivors which bore tumors. The reduction in tumor incidence was most clearly evident for sites in which the "spontaneous" tumor incidence is normally high in the strain of Swiss mice used for the study. The liver was one of these sites. Table II summarizes the data. Sur-

TABLE I

EFFECT OF CONCENTRATIONS OF GROUND NUT OIL ON INCIDENCE OF LIVER CELL TUMORS IN C57BL MICE[a]

Parameter	Sex			
	♂	♂	♀	♀
Ground nut oil in diet (%)	5	10	5	10
Number of mice	80	105	80	105
Survivors to 80 weeks (%)	80	67	93	78
Survivors with one or more histologically "type 2" liver nodules (%)	8	16	7	34
Survivors with one or more histologically malignant liver cell tumors[b] (%)	3	1	1	9

[a]Data from Gellatly (1975).

[b]Gellatly includes both hyperplastic and benign neoplastic lesions within his category of "type 2 nodules."

vival was consistently better in restricted compared with *ad libitum*-fed animals in both sexes and for both of the diets. When the tumor incidence data for the two sexes and for both the diets were combined, the effect of diet restriction in reducing tumor incidence in survivors was highly statistically significant (survivors with one or more neoplasm at any site, $p < .001$; survivors with malignant neoplasm at any site, $p < .01$; survivors with one or more benign or malignant liver cell tumors, $p < .0001$).

These impressive effects of dietary intake on the incidence of liver cell tumors in mice are, in fact, much larger than those of some test chemicals which have come to be labeled as carcinogens as a consequence of enhancement of liver tumor incidence in mice. The situation would, thus, seem to be wide open for the generation of both false-positive and false-negative results. A true liver carcinogen that reduces appetence might theoretically reduce overall tumor incidence, and even specifically liver tumor incidence, more by reducing food intake than it increases it because of its hepatocarcinogenic activity. Alternatively, a test chemical that increases appetence and food intake (e.g., sucrose—Hunter *et al.*, 1978) may increase liver tumor incidence nonspecifically. Another potential problem relates to the use of oily vehicles in carcinogenicity tests involving exposure via gavage. Oil given in this way may profoundly alter the nutritional status of

TABLE II

EFFECT OF DIET RESTRICTION ON SURVIVAL, INCIDENCE OF TUMORS AT ANY SITE, AND ON LIVER TUMOR INCIDENCE IN SWISS MICE[a]

	Diet 1 (PRD)[b]				Diet 2 (41B)[b]			
	♂		♀		♂		♀	
	AL	75%	AL	75%	AL	75%	AL	75%
Number of mice	80	80	80	80	80	80	80	80
Survival for 18 months (%)	60	69	60	80	56	64	64	74
Survivors with one or more neoplasms of any kind (%)	40**[c]	15	25**	6	62**	31	27	14
Survivors with one or more malignant neoplasms of any kind (%)	8	2	6	2	9	2	12	5
Survivors with one or more liver cell tumors (%)	23**	4	4	2	47***	12	6	0

[a]From Conybeare (1980).
[b]AL, *Ad libitum;* 75%, 75% of *ad libitum.*
[c]**AL > Restricted, $p < .01$; ***AL > Restricted, $p < .001$.

animals. It is very easy for experimentalists to forget that a dose of 0.1 ml oil to a 25-g mouse is equivalent, on a body weight basis, to a dose of over 250 ml oil to an adult human!

It should not, however, be assumed that excessive caloric intake is the sole determinant of the effect of overnutrition in increasing liver cell tumor incidence in mice. In rats, overnutrition causes a wide spectrum of endocrine imbalances. It is possible, therefore, that the effect of overnutrition on liver tumor risk in mice is hormone-mediated. The fact that male mice are more susceptible than females to the "spontaneous development" of liver cell tumors is consistent with there being a hormonal influence on liver tumor risk. Also of possible importance is the fact that, under conditions of diet restriction, animals spend some part of each day with an empty, bacteriologically sterile stomach and small intestine, whereas under conditions of continuous availability of food, there may be no period of the day in which upper gastrointestinal bacterial sterility exists.

At present, the precise explanation of how overnutrition enhances liver tumor risk in mice remains unclear and in urgent need of elucidation.

D. Partial Hepatectomy, Necrosis, and Regeneration

In rats, carefully timed partial hepatectomy enhances liver tumor incidence where there is concomitant exposure to known liver carcinogens (Craddock, 1977; Tatematsu *et al.*, 1977). Whether the same is true for mice and other species has not been adequately researched.

In mice, there is considerable circumstantial evidence for a threshold dose level for enhancement of liver cell tumor risk from exposure to nonmutagenic hepatotoxins (such as carbon tetrachloride, chloroform, and selenium), which relates to the dose required to cause repeated cycles of liver cell necrosis followed by regeneration (Edwards and Dalton, 1942; Eschenbrenner and Miller, 1945; Reitz *et al.*, 1980; FDA, 1974; Jorgenson *et al.*, 1985).

Other work suggests that liver cell injury which is not severe enough to result in necrosis may also contribute to liver cell tumor risk. This sequence of events has been described for nonmutagenic chemicals such as Ponceau MX and safrole (Crampton *et al.*, 1977; Grasso and Gray, 1977; Grasso, 1979).

E. Liver Enlargement Associated with Disturbed Lysosomal Pattern and Peroxisomal Proliferation

Some, but not all, hypolipidemic and porphyria-inducing agents and the phthalates cause enlargement of the liver and ultrastructural evidence of lysosomal disturbance and peroxisomal proliferation, but no overt evidence of liver cell damage in short-term tests. In the long term these same, nonmutagenic agents enhance liver tumor incidence in rats (Cohen and Grasso, 1981; De Matteis, 1978; NTP, 1982). More information with regard to the nongenotoxic mechanism involved in liver tumorigenesis by agents which cause these ultrastructural changes is needed. However, one fact seems clear: mere liver enlargement by itself is of limited value for the prediction of increased tumor risk. In the case of agents which stimulate peroxisomal proliferation, liver enlargement is associated with increased risk of subsequent liver tumor development. In the absence of significant increased liver weight, liver tumor risk is not enhanced by such agents. On the other hand, the rodent liver increases two- or threefold during pregnancy as a physiological adaptive change (Wilson *et al.*, 1970). This enlargement is not associated with increased liver tumor risk.

F. The Role of Increased Metabolic Activity and/or Cell Turnover

The link between the several nongenotoxic factors which enhance liver cell tumorigenesis may simply be an increased rate of metabolic activity within liver cells and/or an increased rate of cell turnover. During ordinary metabolic processes numerous electrophilic metabolites capable of damaging cell proteins including DNA are formed. Overnutrition and various forms of metabolic stress may lead to increased cellular and nuclear damage as a result of increased production of endogenously generated electrophiles (Ames, 1983). Also, or alternatively, if there is a risk of genetic error during cell replication, then the rate of accumulation of such errors in liver cells is likely to depend on the rate of liver cell replication. In this way, nongenotoxins which nonspecifically enhance some aspect of cellular metabolic activity and/or the rate of cell turnover may indirectly predispose to the accumulation of genetic damage (i.e., because they increase free-radical production), leading to increased cancer risk. Relevant to this theory is the fact that increase in peroxisome numbers is associated with inceased hydrogen peroxide-generating oxidases and long-chain fatty acid oxidation enzymes (Reddy and Krishnakantha, 1975; Osumi and Hashimoto, 1979). High-fat diets also give rise to peroxisomal proliferation with increased peroxisomal β-oxidation (Ishii *et al.*, 1980; Neat *et al.*, 1980).

VI. The Significance of Enzyme-Altered Foci in the Pathogenesis of Hepatocellular Neoplasia

During recent years, there has been an increasing interest in the observation that agents which give rise to liver cell tumors in rodents in the long term often give rise to a wide variety of enzyme-altered liver cell foci in the short term (Gossner and Friedrich-Freksa, 1964; Friedrich-Freksa *et al.*, 1969a,b; Schauer and Kunze, 1968; Schieferstein *et al.,* 1974; Scherer and Emmelot, 1976; Sirica *et al.,* 1978). Among the enzyme alterations most studied are (1) absent glucose-6-phosphatase, (2) absent ATPase, (3) diminished glycogen phosphorylase, (4) elevated arylesterase, (5) elevated β-glutamyl transpeptidase, (6) elevated epoxide hydrolase. A real insight into the nature of these localized liver changes might throw useful light not only on the pathogenesis of hepatocellular neoplasia but also, more generally, on the mechanisms of all forms of carcinogenesis. It is rightly or wrongly assumed that the foci represent clones of altered cells with each clone being derived from a single altered cell. The first question, therefore, concerns the nature of the cellular alteration. Is it a consequence of a change in the genetic information within the cell or merely a phenotypic expressional change (Pitot *et al.,* 1974)? The fact that liver cells look alike under the microscope does not necessarily mean that they are functionally identical. Do islands arise because a subset of the liver cell population respond to a particular metabolic requirement when other cells do not? Is the development of islands simply an adaptive change? There is plenty of evidence that most islands disappear after cessation of exposure to the agent which led to their appearance. However, this does not mean that individual cells returned to normal. More probably, enzyme-altered cells die off rather than divide after exposure ceases or when their purpose, if they have one, has been served. Sequential pathology studies prove that, at most, only a very small minority of islands persist and possibly progress to nodules or actual tumors. Alternatively, the observed facts are consistent with the possibility that no foci of altered hepatocytes progress to neoplasia and that tumors, when they arise, do so de novo from cells that have not passed through a stage of enzyme alteration.

The concept that there is a link between enzyme-island induction and hepatocarcinogenesis is enhanced by the fact that partial hepatectomy increases the incidence of enzyme-altered foci in rats exposed to hepatocarcinogens (Laib and Bolt, 1980; Pitot, 1979). The higher sensitivity of newborn rats, as compared with adult rats, to the induction of enzyme-altered foci in response to hepatocarcinogens ia also consistent with there being a link between island induction and hepatocarcinogenesis. Studies with tritiated thymidine carried out by Scherer and Hoffmann (1971) indicated a faster rate of cell turnover in enzyme-altered foci than in normal liver tissue in rats exposed to diethylnitrosamine.

Altered enzyme foci are not frequently found in untreated rats, particularly with increasing age (Ogawa *et al.,* 1981).

VII. The Prediction of Hepatocarcinogenic Risk for Man

In 1982, the European Chemical Industry Ecology and Toxicology Centre in Brussels assembled a group of scientists, including myself, to produce a monograph entitled "Hepatocarcinogenesis in Laboratory Rodents: Relevance for Man" (ECETOC, 1982). The task of the group was to review the available scientific evidence and to assess the relevance for man of the laboratory data. I have freely drawn on my experience as a member of that group of scientists in preparing the present chapter. I can now do no better than reproduce *Section G* of the report which we prepared. Section G is headed "Sequence of Steps Recommended for Establishing the Hepatocarcinogenic Potential of a Chemical to Laboratory Animals and Man." It is given in Table III (see also Figs. 1 and 2).

VIII. Summary

1. Man is a poor model for the prediction of agents that are hepatocarcinogenic for laboratory rodents. Relatively few agents are known to cause any form of primary liver cancer in man. The most important is hepatitis B virus, for which there is possibly a model in the woodchuck but not one in rats or mice. The only other agents known to cause primary liver cancer in man are certain steroid hormones, vinyl chloride, and thorium dioxide. There are animal models for the first two of these and a reasonable expectation that thorium dioxide would produce liver tumors in animals if the appropriate experiments were done. Aflatoxin, a potent hepatocarcinogen in rats and other species but not mice, is strongly suspected of being an important human hepatocarcinogen in certain geographical areas of the world, but the evidence is circumstantial. There is no more than a weak association between the nutritional type of cirrhosis secondary to excessive intake of alcohol and increased primary liver cancer in man, and no evidence at all that ethanol per se causes liver tumors in mice, rats, hamsters, or mastomys.

2. By contrast, a very large number of chemicals to which people in the West have been exposed for many decades have been found to be hepatocarcinogens in laboratory rodents. In most cases the levels of exposure required to produce liver tumors in rodents far exceed those to which man is normally exposed. The problem is to guess whether low-level exposure to such rodent hepatocarcinogens poses any real liver cancer threat to man?

TABLE III

SEQUENCE OF STEPS RECOMMENDED FOR ESTABLISHING THE HEPATOCARCINOGENIC POTENTIAL OF A CHEMICAL TO LABORATORY ANIMALS AND MAN[a]

The detection of hepatocarcinogenicity relies on long-term studies in animals. Although there are no reliable short-term tests that relate specifically to the detection of hepatocarcinogenicity, an early indication of possible hepatocarcinogenicity, or the lack of it, can be deduced from the results of other tests. Thus, a compound is unlikely to be a hepatocarcinogen if it gives negative results in mutation tests and no liver enlargement or disturbance of liver microarchitecture in an appropriate 14-day rat study. More substantial evidence is the failure to observe adverse hepatic changes in a 90-day rodent study. If liver changes are present in either a 14- or 90-day experiment, they may require further investigation.

1. *Stepwise Approach to the Investigation of Possible Hepatocarcinogenicity.* The sequence of steps is summarized in Figs. 1 and 2. It is emphasized that this guidance scheme should not be interpreted rigidly. The investigations carried out will vary from chemical to chemical, and many factors (e.g., physicochemical properties, potential routes of exposure) may influence the choice of experimental systems.

. . . The first three types of information concern chemical reactivity, genotoxicity, and short-term *in vivo* toxicity studies for identifying possible target tissues and demonstrating the presence or absence of cumulative toxicity. In the light of this information one of the following four positions may be reached (see also Fig. 1):

—Mutation negative, liver changes absent
—Mutation positive, liver changes absent
—Mutation positive, liver changes present
—Mutation negative, liver changes present

When mutagenicity tests are negative, and there is no evidence of hepatotoxicity in short-term tests, then no priority need be given to the investigation of hepatocarcinogenicity.

If mutation tests are positive but there is no evidence of liver toxicity, the next step is to seek confirmation of the mutagenic properties (ECETOC, 1980), possibly extending the search to an investigation of DNA-adduct formation and the nature and response of DNA repair processes. If these mutation tests confirm that the chemical has mutagenic potential, further studies (possibly including long-term animal studies) relevant to possible human exposure will usually be required to assess the carcinogenic potential for organs other than the liver.

If the mutation tests are positive and there is evidence of liver toxicity in short-term tests, corroborative tests for mutagenicity are required (ECETOC, 1980) and short-term toxicity studies extending to other animal species are advisable. These should include interspecies comparative studies to resolve possible variations in qualitative and/or quantitative metabolism and detoxification, including investigations in a nonrodent species. This would aid in the differentiation of species specificity regarding hepatic response. It should not be assumed at this stage that there is any relationship between positive findings in the mutagenicity tests and hepatotoxicity.

If the mutation tests are negative and liver toxicity positive, attempts should be made to confirm nongenotoxicity using a relevant *in vivo* procedure (ECETOC, 1980). The nature of the hepatotoxicity should also be characterized. Possible observations may include classical histopathological changes (e.g. zonal/focal degeneration) in the absence

(*continued*)

Table III (*Continued*)

of liver enlargement, in which instance the compound is a hepatotoxin and attempts at determining no-effect levels should be made. Alternatively, liver enlargement may be observed in the absence of histopathological changes, and in this situation attempts should be made to differentiate between liver cell enlargement *per se* and cell proliferation. Studies such as thymidine incorporation, estimation of ploidy, and counting of mitotic figures are useful in differentiating between the two processs. In many cases both cell enlargement and cell proliferation may be observed. Where cell proliferation is encountered, the use of other rodent or nonrodent species should be considered to give a better asessment of potential human hazard.

Cell enlargement is frequently encountered and can be detected by microscopic or biochemical (DNA concentration) procedures. Factors often responsible for liver cell enlargement are increased intracellular lipid, or the proliferation of peroxisomes and smooth endoplasmic reticulum. Fatty infiltration may be determined histochemically, while proliferation of subcellular organelles may be measured either ultrastructurally or biochemically. Peroxisome proliferation may at times be preceded by fatty change of the liver, and hence if lipid accumulation is observed one might look carefully for peroxisome proliferation at a later stage.

There seems to be little, if any, causal relationship between the proliferation of smooth endoplamic reticulum (SER) and hepatocarcinogenicity. Conversely, there seems to be a reasonably good correlation between the ability of a chemical to elicit peroxisome proliferation and the subsequent appearance of hepatic tumors in rodents. To assess the significance of such observations for man, short-term *in vivo* tests in a nonrodent species should be considered.

2. *The Importance of Comparative Studies of Metabolism and Pharmacokinetics.* Much of the above is relevant to the question of extrapolation to man. However, the most important information for genotoxic and nongenotoxic carcinogens alike comes from comparative studies of metabolism and pharmacokinetics. In the biotransformation of exogenous chemicals there can be important qualitative as well as quantitative differences between species and it is essential in assessing the possibility or extent of adverse effects in man, to look for such differences and take account of them.

[a]Extract from ECETOC (1982).

3. The mortality from primary liver cancer is very low in countries such as England and Wales where there is widespread exposure to low doses of both natural and synthetic agents which, in high dosage, cause liver tumors in rodents. This suggests that, if there is any risk, it can only be very small.

4. Death rate data collected in England and Wales by the Registrar General are consistent with there having been a small increase in the incidence of primary liver cancer in England and Wales during the past 20 years, but the apparent increase might well be a consequence of revisions in the International Classification of Diseases system and not real. During the first half of the present century the age-standard-

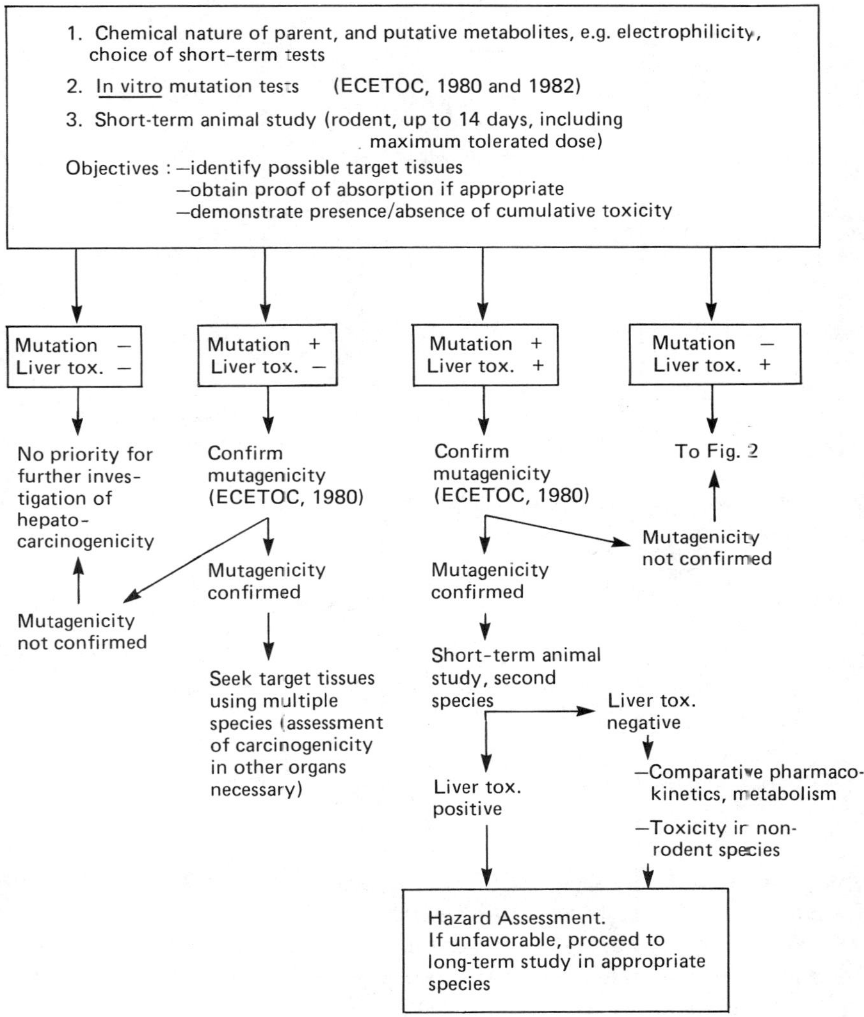

FIG. 1. Sequence of steps—I.

ized incidence of primary liver cancer in England and Wales was falling.

5. In all species, agents which cause liver necrosis with subsequent regeneration and the development of macronodular cirrhosis should probably be suspected of increasing the liver cancer risk, possibly by

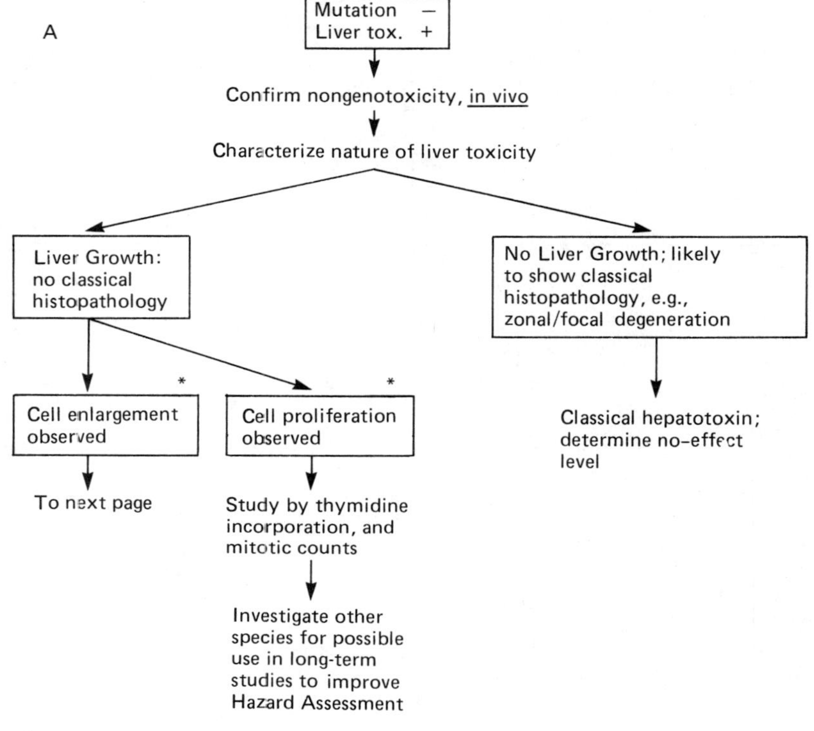

FIG. 2. Sequence of steps—II.

what has been referred to as a "tumor-promoting" process, although the use of this latter term is questioned.

6. The effect of partial hepatectomy in enhancing the hepatocarcinogenic effect of other agents is, perhaps, equivalent to the enhancing effect of regenerative hyperplasia.

7. Agents which in high dosages over long periods give rise to primary liver tumors in rodents give rise to a *variety* of changes after shorter periods of exposure to the same agents. This suggests that there may be many alternative pathways from normal to neoplasia.

8. Neither for man nor for rodents is it certain whether primary liver cancers can develop in the absence of preceding detectable liver damage. However, in tests in which rodents develop liver tumors following exposure to high doses of xenobiotic agents, it is rare for there to be no evidence of previous and/or contemporary liver damage.

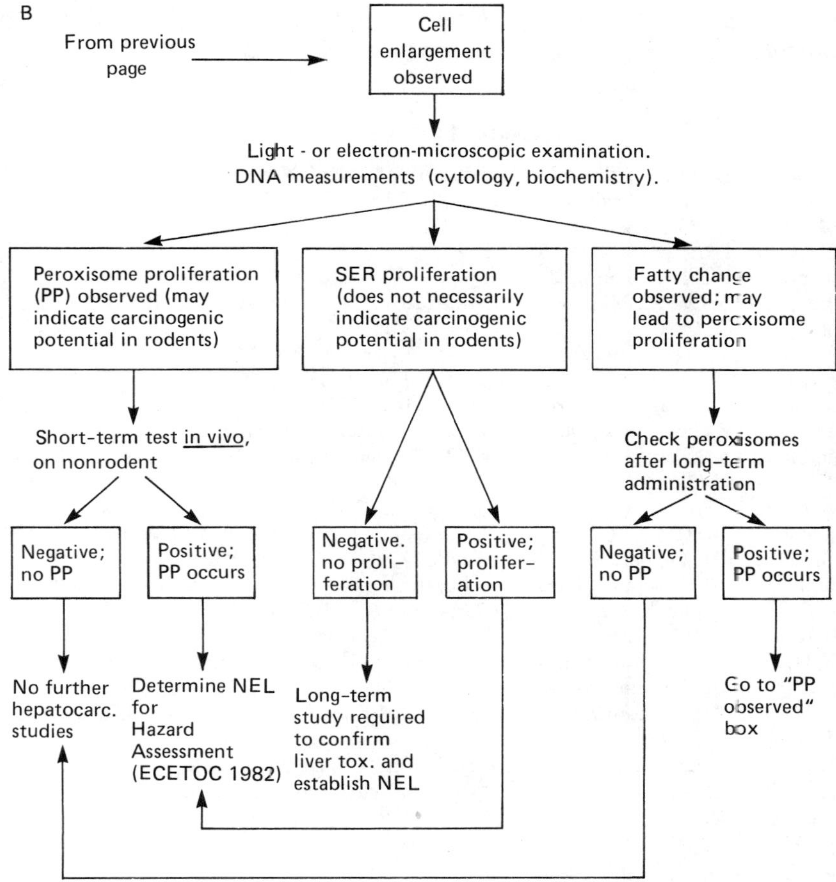

FIG. 2. (*Continued*)

Therefore, there is much to be said for attempting to obtain a better insight into the liver changes which precede liver cancer development in rodents and to develop sensitive, noninvasive, tests for ascertaining whether exposed humans show similar hepatic changes.

9. On the basis of present knowledge, agents which cause liver tumors in rodents by a genotoxic mechanism merit more concern than those that do so by a nongenotoxic mechanism. Features for distinguishing between these two kinds of mechanisms are discussed.

10. In the light of the data reviewed, mathematical calculations of liver tumor risk to humans based on tumor data derived from rodent

studies exposed to very high doses are wholly unreliable both from a qualitative and a quantitative viewpoint.

References

Adamson, R. H., Correa, P., and Dalgard, D. W. (1973). *J. Natl. Cancer Inst.* **50,** 549–553.

Agnew, L. R. C., and Gardner, W. V. (1952). *Cancer Res.* **12,** 757.

Ames, B. N. (1983). *Science* **221,** 1256–1264.

Andervont, H. B. (1950). *J. Natl. Cancer Inst.* **11,** 581.

Andervont, H. B., and Dunn, T. B. (1962). *J. Natl. Cancer Inst.* **28,** 1153–1163.

Arrigoni, A., Zago, P., Mazzucco, D., Andriulli, A., and Rizzetto, M. (1985). *Lancet,* **2,** 277.

Baum, J. K., Holtz, F., Bookstein, J. J., and Kleine, E. W. (1973). *Lancet* **2,** 926.

Boyd, J. T., Langlands, A. O., and Maccabe, J. J. (1968). *Br. Med. J.* **2,** 517–521.

Case, R. A. M. (1956). *Br. J. Prev. Soc. Med.* **10,** 172–199.

Cohen, J., and Grasso, P. (1981). *Food Cosmet. Toxicol.* **19,** 585.

Committee on Safety of Medicines (1972). "Carcinogenicity Tests of Oral Contraceptives." Her Majesty's Stationery Office, London.

Conybeare, G. (1980). *Food Cosmet. Toxicol.* **18,** 65–75.

Craddock, V. M. (1977). *In* "Primary Liver Tumours" (H. Remmer, H. M. Bolt, P. Bannasch, and H. Popper, eds.), pp. 30 and 377. M.T.P. Press. Lancaster.

Crampton, R. F., Gray, T. J., Grasso, P., and Parke, D. V. (1977). *Toxicology* **7,** 307.

Creech, J. L., and Johnson, M. N. (1974). *J. Occup. Med.* **16,** 150.

De Matteis, F. (1978). *Pharmacol. Ther. Part A* **2,** 693.

ECETOC (1980). A Contribution to the Strategy for the Identification and Control of Occupational Carcinogens. Monograph No. 2.

ECETOC (1982). Hepatocarcinogenesis in Laboratory Rodents: Relevance for Man. Monograph No. 4.

Edwards, J. E., and Dalton, A. J. (1942). *J. Natl. Cancer Inst.* **3,** 19.

Eschenbrenner, A. B., and Miller, E. (1945). *J. Natl. Cancer Inst.* **5,** 251.

Farrell, G. C., Joshua, D. E., Uren, R. F., Baird, P. J., Perkus, K. W., and Kronenberg, H. (1975). *Lancet* **1,** 430.

F.D.A. (1974). *Fed. Regist.* **39,** 1355.

Friedrich-Freksa, H., Gossner, W., and Borner, P. (1969a). *Z. Krebsforsch.* **72,** 226.

Friedrich-Freksa, H., Papadopulu, G., and Gossner, W. (1969b). *Z. Krebsforsch.* **72,** 240.

Gellatly, J. B. M. (1975). *In* "Mouse Hepatic Neoplasia" (W. H. Butler and P. M. Newberne, eds.), pp. 77–109. Elsevier, Amsterdam.

Gibel, W. (1967). *Arch. Geschwülstforsch.* **30,** 181–189.

Goodman, D. G., Ward, J. M., Squire, R. A., Chu, K. C., and Linhart, M. S. (1979). *Toxicol. Appl. Pharmacol.* **48,** 237.

Gossner, von, W., and Friedrich-Freksa, H. (1964). *Z. Naturforsch.* **19b,** 862.

Grasso, P. (1979). *Arch. Toxicol. Suppl.* **2,** 171.

Grasso, P., and Gray, T. J. B. (1977). *Toxicology* **7,** 327.

Grasso, P., and Hardy, J. (1975). *In* "Mouse Hepatic Neoplasia" (W. H. Butler and P. M. Newberne, eds.), pp. 111–132. Elsevier, Amsterdam.

Herrold, K. McD. (1969). *Br. J. Cancer* **23,** 655–660.

Heston, W. E. (1963). *J. Natl. Cancer Inst.* **31,** 467.

Hollander, C. F., and Higginson, J. (1971). *J. Natl. Cancer Inst.* **46,** 1343–1355.

Hunter, B., Graham, C., Heywood, R., Prentice, D., and Magnusson, C. (1978). Huntingdon Research Centre Report No. HLR7/7729.
Ishii, H., Fukumori, N., Horie, S., and Suga, T. (1980). *Biochim. Biophys. Acta* **617,** 1.
Johnson, F. L., Feagler, J. R., and Lerner, K. W. (1972). Association of androgenic-anabolic steroid therapy with development of hepatocellular carcinoma. *Lancet* **2,** 1273.
Johnson, P. J., and Williams, R. (1972). *Br. Med. J.* **284,** 1586.
Jorgenson, T. A., Meierhenry, E. F., Rushbrook, C. J., Bull, R. J., and Robinson, M. (1985). *Fundam. Appl. Toxicol.* **5,** 760–769.
Ketcham, A. S., Wexler, H., and Mantel, N. (1963). *Cancer Res.* **23,** 667–670.
Kraybill, H. F., and Shimkin, M. B. (1964). *Adv. Cancer Res.* **8,** 191–248.
Kuratsune, M., Kohchi, S., Horie, A., and Nishizumi, M. (1971). *Gann* **62,** 395–405.
Laib, R. J., and Bolt, H. M. (1980). *Verh. Dtsch. Ges. Arbeitsmed.* **20,** 537.
Lancaster, M. C., Jenkins, F. P., and Philp, J. M. (1961). *Nature (London)* **192,** 1095.
Larouze, B., London, W. T., Saimot, G., Werner, H. G., Lustbader, E. D., Payet, M., and Blumberg, B. S. (1976). *Lancet* **II,** 534.
Lee, F. I. (1966). *Gut* **7,** 77.
Linsell, C. A. (1978). *Proc. Int. Cancer Congr., 12th* **IX,** Digestive Cancer.
Maclure, K. M., and MacMahon, B. (1980). *Epdiemiol. Rev.* **2,** 19–48.
MacMahon, H. E., Murphy, A. S., and Bates, M. I. (1947). *Am. J. Pathol.* **23,** 585.
Maltoni, C. (1977). *In* "Origins of Human Cancer" (H. H. Hiatt, J. D. Watson, and J. A. Winsten, eds.), Book A, pp. 119–146. Cold Spring Harbor Laboratory, Cold Spring Harbor, New York.
Neat, C. E., Thomassen, M. S., and Osmundsen, H. (1980). *Biochem. J.* **186,** 369.
Nettleship, A., and Fink, W. J. (1961). *Am. J. Clin. Pathol.* **35,** 422–426.
Neuberger, J., Portmann, B., Nunnerley, H. B., Laws, J. W., Davis, M., and Williams, R. (1980). *Lancet* **1,** 273.
NTP—National Toxicology Programme (1982). *NIH Publ.* 82–1773.
Ogawa, K., Onoe, T., and Takeuchi, M. (1981). *J. Natl. Cancer Inst.* **67,** 407.
Osumi, T., and Hashimoto, T. (1979). *J. Biochem. (Tokyo)* **85,** 131.
Pitot, H. C. (1979). *In* "The Induction of Drug Metabolism" (R. W. Estabrook and E. Lindenlaub, eds.), p. 471. Schattauer, Stuttgart.
Pitot, H. C., Shirer, T., Moore, E., and Garrett, G. T. (1974). *In* "Molecular Biology of Cancer" (H. Busch ed.), p. 513. Academic Press, New York.
Prince, A. M. (1981). *Hepatology* **1,** 73.
Reddy, J. K., and Krishnakantha, T. P. (1975). *Science* **190,** 787.
Reddy, J. K., and Svoboda, D. J. (1975). *Fed. Proc., Fed. Am. Soc. Exp. Biol.* **34,** 827.
Registrar-General (1978). "Decennial Supplement on Occupational Mortality in England and Wales 1970–72." Her Majesty's Stationery Office, London.
Reitz, R. H., Quast, J. F., Stott, W. T., Watanabe, P. G., and Gehring, P. J. (1980). *In* "Water Chlorination, Environmental Impact and Health Effects" (R. L. Jolley, W. H. Bungs, and R. B. Cummings, eds.), Vol. 3, p. 983. Ann Arbor Science Publ., Ann Arbor, Michigan.
Rowlatt, C., Franks, L. M., and Sheriff, M. U. (1973). *Br. J. Cancer* **28,** 83
Schauer, A., and Kunze, E. (1968). Enzymhistochemisches und autoradiographische Untersuchungen während Cancerisierung der Rattenleber mit Diäthylnitrosamin. *Z. Krebsforsch.* **70,** 252.
Scherer, E., and Emmelot, P. (1976). *Cancer Res.* **36,** 2544.
Scherer, E., and Hoffman, M. (1971). *Eur. J. Cancer* **7,** 369.

Schieferstein, G., Pirschel, J., Frank, W., and Friedrich-Freksa, H. (1974). Quantitativ Untersuchungen über den irreversiblen Verlust zweier Enzymativitäten in der Rattenleber nach Verfütterung von Diäthylnitrosamin. *Z. Krebsforsch.* **82,** 191.

Schmahl, D. (1976). *Cancer Lett.* **1,** 215–218.

Shafritz, D. A., and Kew, M. C. (1981). *Hepatology* **I,** 1.

Sinnhuber, R. O., Wales, J. H., Ayres, J. L., Engebrecht, R. H., and Amend, D. L. (1968). *J. Natl. Cancer Inst.* **41,** 711–718.

Sirica, A. E., Barsness, L., Goldworthy, T., and Pitot, H. C. (1978). *J. Environ. Pathol. Toxicol.* **2,** 21.

Sokoloff, L., Mickelsen, O., Silverstein, E., Jay, G. E., Jr., and Yamamoto, R. S. (1960). *Am. J. Physiol.* **198,** 765.

Stemmermann, G. N. (1960). *Am. J. Clin. Pathol.* **34,** 446–454.

Stuart, H. L. (1965). "Geographic Distribution of Hepatic Cancer in Primary Hepatoma" (W. J. Burdette, ed.). Univ. of Utah Press, Salt Lake City.

Summers, J. (1981). *Hepatology* **I,** 179.

Swarm, R. K., Miller, E., and Michelitch, H. J. (1962). *Pathol. Microbiol.* **25,** 27–44.

Sweeney, E. C., and Evans, D. J. (1976). *J. Clin. Pathol.* **29,** 626.

Tannenbaum, A. (1940). *Am. J. Cancer* **38,** 335.

Tannenbaum, A. (1947). *Ann. N.Y. Acad. Sci.* **49,** 5.

Tannenbaum, A., and Silverstone, H. (1949). *Cancer Res.* **9,** 162.

Tatematsu, M., Shirai, T., Tsuda, H., Miyata, Y., Shinohara, Y., and Ito, N. (1977). *Gann* **68,** 499.

Thompson, J. G. (1961). Primary carcinoma of the liver in the three ethnic groups in Capetown, *Acata,* U.I.C.C. **17,** 632.

Tuyns, A. J. (1979). *Cancer Res.* **39,** 2840–2843.

Vesselinovitch, S. D., Mihailovich, N., Wogan, G. N., Lombard, L. S., and Rao, K. V. N. (1972). *Cancer Res.* **32,** 2289–2291.

Wales, J. H., and Sinnhuber, R. O. (1972). *J. Natl. Cancer Inst.* **48,** 1529–1530.

Wilson, R., Doell, B. H., Groger, W., Hope, J., and Gellatly, J. B. M. (1970). *In* "Metabolic Aspects of Food Safety" (F. J. C. Roe, ed.), p. 363. Blackwell, Oxford.

Wogan, G. N. (1969). *Prog. Exp. Tumor Res. (Basel)* **11,** 134–162.

Wogan, G. N., Paglialunga, S., and Newberne, P. M. (1974). *Food Cosmet. Toxicol.* **12,** 681–685.

Neurobehavioral Toxicology: An Overview

DAVID L. HOPPER

Veterinary Diagnostic Laboratory, College of Veterinary Medicine, Iowa State University, Ames, Iowa 50011

I. Introduction

It is well established that the central nervous system (CNS) is essential to the production of behavior. It is equally evident that human and animal behavior can be altered by a variety of chemicals. However, only recently have behavioral measures been recognized as essential in assessing the potential toxicity of these agents to the CNS. This recognition has fostered a new area of research within toxicology which has been referred to by Weiss and Laties (1969) as "behavioral toxicology" and by Zbinden (1983) as "neurobehavioral toxicology." Affirmation of the rapid development of this area of research to the status of a subdiscipline within the field of toxicology comes from the numerous books, book chapters, reviews, and symposia devoted to this subject (Anger and Johnson, 1985; Bigami, 1976; Brimblecombe, 1968, 1976; Evans and Weiss, 1978; Geller *et al.*, 1979; Hopper, 1985; Mello, 1975; Mitchell, 1978, 1982; Mitchell and Tilson, 1982; NIMH, 1984; NAS, 1975, 1977; Norton, 1982; NRC, 1984; Reiter, 1978; Ruffin, 1963; Russell and Singer, 1982; Silverman, 1974; Tilson and Mitchell, 1984; Weiss and Laties, 1969, 1975; Xintaras *et al.*, 1974; Xintaras and Johnson, 1976; Zbinden *et al.*, 1983; Zenick and Reiter, 1977).

The purposes of this review are to define this new subdiscipline of toxicology, examine the rationale for studying the effects of toxicants on behavioral processes, discuss the special significance of animal models in neurobehavioral toxicology, briefly review the historical development of this area of research, examine test methods and some of the variables and conditions affecting their use, discuss the value of corroborating tests, and survey the neurotoxins of current interest.

Finally, some conjectures as to topics likely to be of significant future interest to neurobehavioral toxicologists are discussed.

A. What Is Neurobehavioral Toxicology?

In attempting to provide an answer to the question, "What is toxicology?" Casarett (1975) noted that despite the simplicity of the question, there is no simple answer and the difficulty in providing an answer is a consequence of the multidisciplinary nature of the field of study. A similar problem exists when attempting to define "behavioral toxicology" or "neurobehavioral toxicology." Using the definition of behavioral pharmacology offered by Thompson and Schuster (1968) as a model, behavioral toxicology can be defined as a branch of biological science that uses the tools and concepts of experimental psychology and toxicology to explore the behavioral actions of toxicants. Some toxicologists argue that the term "behavioral toxicology" is too restrictive and does not reflect important aspects of work in this subdiscipline of toxicology. In a discussion of the meaning of the term "neurobehavioral toxicology," Zbinden (1983) emphasized that toxicologists not only study functional changes in the nervous system but morphological and biochemical changes as well. Given this, Zbinden contends that the term neurobehavioral toxicology better describes the discipline by reflecting its multidisciplinary nature. Neurobehavioral toxicology might be defined as a branch of biological science that uses the methods and concepts of experimental psychology and toxicology to explore the behavioral actions of toxicants and the methods and concepts of other disciplines to investigate associated nonbehavioral toxicant-related changes. Typically, nonbehavioral changes include those which might be referred to as biochemical, morphological, or physiological. In an effort to acknowledge the multidisciplinary nature of this subdiscipline of toxicology, the term "neurobehavioral toxicology" will be used in this chapter.

B. Rationale for the Study of Neurobehavioral Toxicology

There are a number of compelling reasons for evaluating behavior when assessing the toxicity of a chemical. A fundamental reason for examining the behavioral effects of toxicants given by Dews and Wenger (1979) is that, at the present level of scientific development, morphological and chemical changes may not be discernible at a time when behavior is profoundly altered. Mello (1975) argues that behavior is the end point of the functional activity of the nervous system and functional capacity cannot be determined independently of behavioral analysis. Norton (1982) points out that behavioral measures assess CNS function and not excess capacity, structural redundancy, or damage for which compensation has occurred. Another compelling reason, particularly for the toxicologist with a behavioral background, is the expectation that neurotoxicants can be used as tools to aid in understanding behavioral phenomena. From a practical viewpoint, behavioral tests are of value in assessing toxicity because they are, for the most part, noninvasive and thereby allow repeated tests in subjects that are free of the confounding conditions often associated with invasive procedures. Many researchers study the behavioral effects of a toxicant along with morphological, physiological, and biochemical effects with the goal of gaining insight into the relationship of behavior to these phenomena. Finally, some neurobehavioral toxicologists optimistically contend that behavioral tests will prove to be more sensitive than other tests in detecting central nervous toxicity. If behavioral tests are found to be more sensitive they will be of value in detecting incipient toxicity at a point when the progress may be reversible.

These are a few of the reasons for evaluating the behavioral effects of toxicants. The critical point is that the hazard evaluation of a potential neurotoxin cannot be considered complete until potential functional effects are assessed (Norton, 1980).

C. Use of Animal Models in Neurobehavioral Toxicology

Many toxicologists argue that the most appropriate subjects from which to obtain neurobehavioral toxicity data are human beings. The latter argument is based upon the assumption that toxicity data are collected for the purpose of preventing toxicoses in humans. To a large extent this argument is true. However, not all neurobehavioral toxicology studies are conducted with the intent of directly determining the effects of toxicants on humans, and for a number of important reasons a comparative approach is frequently used to study the neurobehavioral effects of toxicants.

One obvious reason for the use of animal models in toxicology research is that for ethical reasons many toxicants or doses of toxicants cannot be administered to human subjects. Although the use of animal model may often not be a matter of choice, in many instances animal models are preferentially selected. Spyker (1974), with specific reference to developmental toxicology studies, reviewed some of the advantages of the use of animal models. Many of these advantages apply equally well to nondevelopmental studies. Some of these advantages are that (1) many animals have short life spans which enable the study of the effects of toxicants from birth to death; (2) environmental and testing conditions can be much more closely controlled for animal than human subjects; (3) when using animals the state of the subject may be altered (lesion, chemical change, disease condition, etc.) to allow testing a hypothesis; (4) it is possible to select animal subjects possessing special attributes or characteristics; and (5) genetic background can be controlled by means of selective breeding, inbreeding, crossbreeding, or mutation.

In addition to providing benefits, the use of animal models in neurobehavioral toxicology or toxicology in general creates a number of problems for the investigator. The majority of these problems are related to extrapolating animal data to the human population. Gehring and Rao (1979) have provided an good review of the problems of extrapolating animal data to humans. Among the more critical problems discussed are the relative sensitivity of the animal model and humans to the toxicant being studied, and the heterogeneity of the human population compared with the animal population studied. These authors point out that species differences in reactions to a given toxicant exposure are generally the result of differences in absorption, distribution, biotransformation, and excretion. Fortunately, species differences in reaction to a toxicant per se at the receptor site are thought to be a rare occurrence.

A cursory search of the neurobehavioral toxicology literature demonstrates that a majority of neurobehavioral toxicology research to date has utilized animal models. For the reasons listed above it is most probable that the use of animal models in toxicology research will increase. As neurobehavioral toxicology grows as a discipline it will become increasingly imperative that extrapolations of neurobehavioral toxicological data to humans from animal models be accomplished with greater reliability. Gehring and Rao (1979) emphasize that greater reliability in extrapolation will come through (1) quantitative knowledge of the absorption, distribution, biotransformation, and excretion of a toxicant or its biotransformation products in humans versus animals, and (2) elucidation of the mechanism of action of the active chemical with the biological receptor. The difficulty of obtaining these data on a significant number of toxicants is acknowledged by these authors, and they suggest that in the near future knowledge of the pharmacokinetic parameters will lead to improvements in extrapolating toxicity data to humans.

II. Neurobehavioral Toxicology: A Historical Perspective

Even a brief review of the literature (Weiss and Laties, 1969, 1975; Xintaras *et al.*, 1974; Xintaras and Johnson, 1976) reveals that neurobehavioral toxicology had its origin, in the United States, predominantly within a few principal areas of endeavor: (1) academic research in pharmacology, specifically psychopharmacology and behavioral pharmacology, (2) industrial and government-sponsored research related to worker safety and the effects of exposure to workplace toxicants, and (3) the research resulting from the legislation enacted in the early 1970s in response to the nationwide concern for the quality of the environment and its effects on the quality of life. The significance of each of these areas to the growth and development of neurobehavioral toxicology are evident from the short historical review that follows.

A. Early Work in Neurobehavioral Toxicology

Beard (1974) traces the development of neurobehavioral toxicology in the United States to the early 1960s and the work of Armstrong *et al.* (1963) at the University of Rochester, Goldberg *et al.* (1962) at the Mellon Institute in Pittsburgh, and his own work (Beard and Wertheim, 1967) at Stanford University. In the late 1960s Van Gelder and his co-workers established a behavioral toxicology laboratory in the College of Veterinary Medicine at Iowa State University and began a series of neurobehavioral toxicological studies in sheep and primates (Sandler *et al., 1968, 1969; Van Gelder et al.*, 1968, 1970, 1973; Van Gelder and Smith, 1973).

One of the earliest references to neurobehavioral toxicology (behavioral toxicology) as an autonomous area of research was made by Weiss and Laties (1969) in their chapter on behavioral pharmacology in the *Annual Review of Pharmacology*. In June 1972 the Department of Radiation Biology and Biophysics at the University of Rochester was the sponsor of the first formal meeting in the United States devoted to behavioral toxicology (Weiss and Laties, 1975). In June of the following year the National Institue for Occupational Safety and Health (NIOSH) and the University of Cincinnati hosted a workshop entitled "The Behavioral Toxicology Workshop for Early Detection of Occupational Hazards." The proceedings of these early meetings gave neurobehavioral toxicology its first books.

Following these early meetings the mid-1970s was a period of further growth and development. In 1976 a symposium entitled, "Behavioral Toxiology: An Emerging Discipline" was sponsored by the Southwest Psychological Association. The proceedings of this meeting resulted in the publication of a third volume exclusively dedicated to the topic of neurobehavioral toxicology (Zenick and Reiter, 1977). In 1979 several significant events in the development of neurobehavioral toxicology occurred. The first of these events was the publication of two new journals: *Neurotoxicology* and *Neurobehavioral Toxicology* (in 1981 *Neurobehavioral Toxicology* was renamed *Neurobehavioral Toxicology and Teratology*). Later in the same year the Southwest Foundation for Research and Education, sponsored by the Office of Toxic Substances of the United States Environmental Protection Agency, organized a workshop entitled "Test Methods for Definition of Effects of Toxic Substances on Behavior and Neuromotor Function." The proceedings of this workshop, which were published as a supplement to *Neurobehavioral Toxicology* (Geller *et al.*, 1979), provided the discipline with another major work. The number of symposia and publications devoted to the area of neurobehavioral toxicology since the late 1970s are too numerous to list in a short review; however, a few of the more important publications are included in the references (see Section I).

B. Federal Legislation and Agencies Important to the Development of Neurobehavioral Toxicology

In the United States the decade of the 1970s, from the perspective of public concern for the environment and governmental response to those concerns, provided many significant contributions to the development of neurobehavioral toxicology. In 1970 Congress enacted the Occupational Safety and Health Act under which the Occupational Safety and Health Administration was formed. Sections 20 and 21 of this act gave the Secretary of Health, Education and Welfare broad authority to conduct experimental research relating to occupational safety and health. Section 22 of the act established the National Institute for Occupational Safety and Health (NIOSH) to implement the provisions of Sections 20 and 21 of the act (Munsch and Potter, 1979). Since its formation NIOSH has taken a very active leadership role in the support and development of neurobehavioral toxicology (Anger, 1984; Anger and Johnson, 1985; Xintaras and Burg, 1980; Xintaras *et al.*, 1974).

In 1970 Congress also enacted the National Environmental Policy Act, which led to the formation of the Environmental Protection Agency (EPA). The Neurotoxicology Division of the Health Effects Research Laboratory at the EPA has, for several years, had an active intramural program of neurobehavioral toxicology research. It has also supported a significant program of extramural research (Geller *et al.*, 1979; Zenick and Reiter, 1977). In 1976 the Toxic Substances Control Act became law. Under the provisions of this act the EPA, which administers the act, is responsible not only for evaluating the teratogenic, mutagenic, and carcinogenic effects of toxic substances, but also behavioral alterations resulting from exposure to these agents (Cabe and Eckerman, 1982; Page, 1979). In addition, the EPA manages several federally legislated programs (The Clean Air Act, 1970; The Federal Water Pollution Control Act, 1972; The Marine Protection Research and Sanctuaries Act, 1972; The Federal Insecticide, Fungicide and Rodenticide Act of 1948, amended in 1972; The Resources Conservation and Recovery Act, 1976) enacted or amended during the 1970s, which have been sources of support for neurobehavioral toxicology research (Reiter, 1980).

In 1978 the National Toxicology Program (NTP) was established as a Department of Health and Human Services (DHHS) cooperative effort to develop information concerning hazardous chemicals, and in 1981 it was given program status. The NTP represents a cooperative effort between several government agencies (the National Cancer Institute, the National Institute of Environmental Health Sciences, the National Center for Toxicological Research, and the National Institute for Occupational Safety and Health) to coordinate research and testing activities concerning toxic chemicals (NTP, 1984). From its inception this program has grown into a major federal resource for toxicity testing. Each year the NTP publishes a detailed annual plan which outlines its program of research. Neurobehavioral toxicology has been, and continues to be, a major research interest of the program. In 1980 the NTP commissioned the National Research Council (NRC) and the National Academy of Sciences to conduct a study to characterize the toxicity testing needs for substances to which there is known or anticipated human exposure, and to develop and validate uniformly applicable and wide-ranging criteria by which to set priorities for research on these substances. The results of this study were recently published

(NRC/NAS, 1984). The procedures outlined in that document for neurobehavioral testing and selecting chemicals for study will undoubtedly have a significant impact on neurobehavioral toxicology research.

III. Methods in Neurobehavioral Toxicology

The methods employed in examining the behavioral effects of toxicants are largely adapted from those used in pharmacology (either behavioral pharmacology or psychopharmacology) (Thompson and Schuster, 1968), experimental psychology (Tilson and Harry, 1982), and ethology (Davis, 1982). A detailed description of the behavioral methods employed in neurobehavioral toxicology will not be given here as several excellent reviews are available (Norton, 1982; Geller *et al.,* 1979; Mitchell, 1982). Methods from a number of other disciplines such as chemistry, physiology, pathology, morphology, and medicine are also employed in neurobehavioral toxicology research (Zenick and Reiter, 1977). For neurobehavioral toxicology the problem has not been one of a lack of methods, but one of (1) determining how most effectively to use available methods so that valid, reliable, cost-effective, and meaningful data are obtained, and (2) understanding and effectively managing a number of conditions and variables that significantly affect experimental results.

A. Methodology: Testing

It is obvious that a variety of chemicals can alter behavior or the functional capacity of the CNS. However, the procedures to be followed in assessing the real or potential risk to CNS function posed by such agents are less obvious. At present, neurobehavioral toxicologists are debating a number of issues concerning test procedures. The issues receiving significant attention are (1) the criteria to use in selecting procedures for evaluating neurobehavioral toxicity, (2) the strategy or strategies to employ in the application of selected tests, and (3) how effectively to screen the enormous number of chemicals to which humans are exposed.

1. Criteria for Test Selection

A number of criteria for the selection of neurobehavioral tests have been proposed; a few of the more important are discussed below.

a. Epidemiology. Tilson and Cabe (1978), Dews and Wenger (1979), and Zbinden (1983) have pointed out the importance of epidemiological data in providing critical information concerning risk assessment and the selection of appropriate neurobehavioral tests. The test procedures used to evaluate the toxicity of a particular agent should, when possible, reflect the signs and symptoms reported by humans exposed to the agent. These data can then be used to select the most relevant procedures for use with animal models, or to direct more comprehensive research with animals without the restrictions imposed by the use of human subjects.

b. Agent. Dews and Wenger (1979) caution against the a priori selection of methods and point out that experience in pharmacology has demonstrated that the agent is a better criterion for evaluation than the test method. Further, these authors state: "If we can agree on agents and loads, than let us each go about assays with all our ingenuity—in the assurance that results will be comparable because of the invariance of agent and load." With the common reference point of the agent, methods can be compared, the better ones selected, and the poorer ones eliminated.

c. Chemical and Physical Change. In a review of methods in behavioral toxicology, Norton (1982) listed several principles on which the function of an organ depends. The first of these principles is that all functional changes are the result of chemical and physical changes in cells. Given this relationship, it is clear that knowledge of the site of action (chemical or physical change) may be of significant value in the selection of neurobehavioral tests by directing attention to tests that purport to measure a function mediated by the affected CNS site. The practical use of physical and chemical cellular changes for test selection is, at present, somewhat limited by the lack of knowledge concerning the functional roles for many of the structures in the CNS.

d. Behavior. Weiss and Laties (1979) propose that aspects of behavior itself be used as the criterion for evaluating neurobehavioral toxicity. Potential neurobehavioral toxicity is determined by tests of a set of functions (behaviors), while the selection of specific tests are left to the discretion of the researcher. This approach allows considerable flexibility in the selection of tests but ensures some commonality via the definition of functions.

e. Validity and Reliability. Tilson and his co-workers (Mitchell and Tilson, 1982; Tilson *et al.*, 1979) and others (Morgan and Repko, 1974; Spyker and Goad, 1983; Zintaras and Johnson, 1976) have been strong advocates for adopting neurobehavioral tests which are sensitive, valid, and reliable. Although taking such a position does not seem particularly unusual, prior to their first publications concerning this issue, the reliability, validity, and reproducibility of neurobehavioral tests was to a large extent ignored. Evans and Weiss (1978) more directly criticized neurobehavioral testing procedures by stating: "Too many studies in behavioral toxicology have been purely descriptive, with neither an attack on underlying mechanisms nor a clear extrapolation to human health questions." To ensure the sensitivity and reliability of neurobehavioral test methods, Tilson *et al.* (1979) recommend that comparisons be made for compounds of known neurotoxic effect using a battery of tests representative of the range of possible functional effects and observed signs and symptoms. Tests are then validated by demonstrating similarities between techniques purporting to measure similar functions or differences between those assumed to measure different processes.

Validity can have several different meanings, and these different meanings have significant implications for neurobehavioral toxicology and merit brief discussion. Validity is a matter of degree rather than an all-or-none property. Validation requires empirical investigations and is an unending process. Simply stated, a measuring instrument (test) is valid if it does what it is intended to do; therefore, one validates not a measuring instrument, but rather a use to which the instrument is put. In the behavioral sciences behavioral measures usually serve three purposes (uses) and each use has a corresponding type of validity: (1) predictive validity, (2) content validity, and (3) construct validity [see Nunnally (1967) for a detailed discussion]. In considering the significance of validity in test selection, Norton (1982) stressed the importance of two aspects of validity, namely, the results of a test should be valid for the species being tested as well as for extrapolation to other species.

A major shortcoming in neurobehavioral toxicology at present is the lack of reliable tests. Reliable tests are tests which produce measures which are repeatable either by the same individual using different measures of the same attribute or by different persons using the same measure of an attribute. It is worthy to note that highly reliable tests are not necessarily highly valid tests. Reliability is a necessary but not sufficient condition for validity, and to this extent these test selection criteria are inextricably linked.

f. Other Criteria. Several other criteria for test selection have been mentioned in the literature. These include the purpose of the study, species, sex, and age (Norton, 1982; Mitchell and Tilson, 1982). Although each of these variables is of obvious importance in test selection, they have not received the attention that the criteria mentioned earlier have.

g. Summary. It is obvious that no single criterion will be adequate for selecting procedures for evaluating the neurobehavioral toxicity of a chemical. Each of the criteria discussed are essential, and each addresses a different aspect of the toxicity testing process. The circumstances surrounding testing will vary for each chemical entity; therefore, it is essential that each of these criteria receive intelligent consideration in the process of determining what methods are to be used.

2. *Strategies for Neurobehavioral Testing*

In addition to the problem of the criteria to use in the selection of neurobehavioral tests, there is the related problem of the strategy to employ in screening chemicals for neurobehavioral toxicity. A number of different screening strategies have been proposed; however, they all share two basic approaches. The first approach employs a single test which is a test generally thought to assess the integrity of a broad range of neural function. The second approach, and clearly the most popular, is some form of sequential testing. Typically this approach utilizes two or more levels of testing with the test results at each level usually having some influence on the tests conducted at subsequent levels.

An example of the first approach is given by Butcher (1976), who discusses the advantages and disadvantages of a single test as a screen for neurobehavioral toxicity. Butcher argues that sensitivity and relevance are the principal attributes of a behavioral test when compared to other procedures (e.g., morphological) for evaluating toxicity. Despite the apparent attractiveness of a single test screen, this approach is subject to a number of difficulties. First, because performance on this type of test typically relies on a number of functional processes, changes in performance cannot be ascribed to a specific functional process (associative, motor, motivational, sensory). Second, a significant functional change in a single functional process may be masked by compensating factors within the same or in other functions. Finally, a single test could not possibly represent the numerous functional capabilities subject to significant toxicological insult. As Stebbins (1982) points out, sophisticated tests designed to answer quantitatively a range of specific questions regarding the continuing changes in health brought on by exposure to toxicants are needed.

The more commonly proposed strategy for neurobehavioral testing is some form of sequential testing. One of the earliest behavioral screening proposals was made in a 1975 National Academy of Science (NAS) report entitled: "Principles for Evaluating Chemicals in the Environment." The screening strategy set forth in this report calls for two levels of tests. The first level is composed of an elementary screen, and the second, a sensitive general behavioral assay. The tests in the elementary screen are crucial to the proposed strategy, for all subsequent behavioral tests depend on a significant finding in the elementary screen. A major criticism of this screening strategy is that significant behavioral changes may go undetected in the elementary screen with the result that tests in the sensitive general behavioral assay would not be conducted.

More recently, Tilson and his co-workers (Tilson *et al.,* 1979, 1980; Mitchell and Tilson, 1982; Mitchell *et al.,* 1982) have proposed a two-level neurobehavioral screening strategy which avoids the strict sequential test dependency of the NAS proposal. Included in the first or preliminary level are tests which provide measures of a broad range of nervous system function (i.e., sensory, motor, arousal, and associative tests). In this proposal the initial behavioral tests are more comprehensive and include tests that are relegated to the secondary screen in the NAS procedures. At present, the tests to be used in the secondary screen have not been specified nor have the criteria for employing these tests. A scenario for such tests will undoubtedly be developed.

Weiss and Laties (1979) oppose the concept of a priori neurobehavioral screening tests. Rather, they propose a functional approach to screening. In this approach the specific behavioral processes to be tested are determined, and the choice of test is left to the investigator. The strategy for screening, with the exception of the functional aspects of behavior to be tested, is completely open. The authors content that such a screening strategy offers many advantages; it would (1) help preclude the adoption of obsolete or inappropriate standards, (2) avoid the waste of resources which would accompany the use of unsuitable standardized tests, (3) promote the development of new test methods, and (4) allow neurobehavioral toxicologists to formulate more adequate and exacting questions.

Dews and Wenger (1979) propose that neurobehavioral toxicity screening should be standardized with respect to agents. The results of screening tests would be comparable because of the invariance provided by the use of specific agents and exposures. The authors propose a three-level screening strategy. Initial screening would employ a simple behavioral test such as a change in spontaneous motor activity (SMA). If changes are observed on the simple test, the agent would be subjected to secondary or even a tertiary level of testing. The goal of the subsequent levels of testing would be to elucidate the mechanism of action. This screening strategy is similar to the NAS proposal in that the initial screen is a simple behavioral test, and subsequent testing is subject to a positive finding on the initial test. Procedures for second- and third-level tests have not been specified.

Reiter *et al.* (1981) have proposed the use of a behavioral toxicity index. The index is based on the acute LD_{50} and experimentally derived ED_{50} values for a range of behavioral tests. A large index value indicates a relatively specific behavioral toxicity and signifies that a behavioral change takes place prior to the onset of overt toxicity. The use of selected behavioral measures to establish a behavioral toxicity index has merit; however, further tests with a number of toxicants are needed before the practicality of the index can be determined.

Although other screening strategies have been proposed (NAS, 1977; Gad, 1981; Pavlenko, 1975; Annau, 1983), the strategies discussed above are representative of the diversity of opinion among behavioral toxicologists concerning how to proceed with neurobehavioral toxicity screening. Although the majority of neurobehavioral toxicologists differ as to the criteria for test selection and strategies for screening, they do agree that neurobehavioral toxicology has not progressed to a point where standardized tests and screening strategies can be locked into regulatory practice. Indeed, many toxicologists contend that to do so would be counterproductive. Given the present status of the discipline, a reasonable approach seems to be to plan research carefully so that critical variables are addressed, and standardize when possible. Through this process the discipline will achieve an information base that will serve as a foundation for future, more comprehensive standardization.

3. *Selecting Chemicals for Study*

If one of the goals of toxicology or neurobehavioral toxicology research is to protect people from toxicological hazard, then chemicals must be tested for potential toxicological effect. According to an estimate based on the Chemical Abstracts Service (CAS) Registry, the number of known chemicals consists of over 5 million entities, and as many as 100,000 chemicals may be in daily use by U.S. industry. As pointed out by Anger (1984), all too often the discovery that a chemical is neurotoxic occurs as a result of unplanned or uncontrolled exposures in an unsuspecting and unintended population. Tilson and Mitchell (1984) point out that the evaluation of all known chemical entities for potential neurobehavioral toxicity is impractical; as a result, there is a need for a well-conceived screening program capable of providing information regarding potential neurotoxicity.

In 1980 the National Toxicology Program (NTP) recognized the need for assessing strategies for selecting chemicals for general toxicological evaluation and issued a contract to the National Research Council (NRC) and NAS to study the problem. The goals for the study were to characterize the toxicity-testing needs for agents to which there is known or anticipated human exposure, and to develop and validate criteria by which to set priorities for research on agents with potential adverse health impact. The results of this study are described in "Toxicity Testing: Strategies to Determine Needs and Priorities" (NRC/NAS, 1984). The study group began its work by examining existing procedures and criteria for determining how chemicals are selected for toxicity evaluation. This review reached the following conclusions: (1) no priority system or screening strategy can be perfect, because the information required for unerring selection is the same as that resulting from the test of every known chemical entity; (2) numerous candidate chemicals must be reduced in number through screening; (3) two principal criteria for screening are estimated human exposure and suspicion of toxicity; and (4) chemicals for which adequate tests have been conducted are of low priority for additional testing. Within government and private institutions, expert judgment has been the traditional means of determining how chemicals are selected for toxicity testing. More recently this process has been supplemented with a variety of analytical techniques. The study group supported the expert-judgment screening strategy as the best strategy given the present limited knowledge concerning chemical hazards. The study group concluded, however, that the current expert-judgment strategy could be improved and suggested two improvements: (1) the value of information concept (the concept asserts that value of information lies in its value in guiding decisions) should be incorporated into priority setting; and (2) a system of validating or checking screening priorities should be established so that the expert-judgment strategy can be improved with accumulated experience.

Anger (1984) discusses the issue of selecting chemicals for study with specific reference to screening workplace chemicals for potential neurotoxicity. Two selection strategies are suggested: (1) exemplars of a structurally related class of chemicals should be studied so that generalizations may be made to the entire class; and (2) chemicals or chemical mixtures actually present in the environment of interest should be evaluated with the goal of identifying general problems. These strategies are to be utilized along with the traditional criteria of the number of individuals exposed and the toxicity of the agent. Anger contends that the employment of these strategies will increase the impact of neurotoxicology research upon regulatory standards.

The strategies discussed above address some of the many facets of this complex issue. Undoubtedly, the enormous number of chemicals, the substantial opportunity for exposure in an industrialized society, and the limited resources for testing will continue to stimulate demands for better tests and selection procedures. Of critical importance is that, regardless of background, neurobehavioral toxicologists continue to evaluate and improve selection strategy.

B. Methodology: Variables and Conditions of Special Concern

There are many variables or conditions which may affect the outcome of a toxicological study, and a few of these are of special concern to neurobehavioral toxicologists.

1. Subject Populations

It can be argued that the most appropriate subjects for neurobehavioral toxicity testing are human beings. However, as a result of moral and ethical considerations, toxicology research with human subjects is often very restricted, thereby necessitating the use of animal models. The selection of an animal model should be based upon toxicological and pharmacological parameters associated with the species chosen for study. For functional studies consideration should also be given to the functional (behavioral) capabilities of the selected species in terms of the behaviors assessed and the hypotheses evaluated. Donovick and Horowitz (1982) discuss the importance of genetic characteristics in the selection of test subjects. Age is often a concern in subject selection as it can have a significant effect on sensitivity to a toxicant, and this is frequently the case for developing organisms and older or senescent animals. For studies at the extremes of the dose–response curve, many subjects will be required to ensure a reasonable probability of detecting response alterations. Finally, practical considerations such as cost, housing, time required for testing, or the availability of test equipment may dictate either the choice of species or the number of subjects.

2. Modifying Attributes of the CNS

Several attributes of the nervous system can significantly modify its response to neurotoxicants. First, some substances capable of entering and affecting tissues of the body are inhibited from entering the brain by the blood–brain barrier (BBB). In the immature CNS the BBB is often less effective, resulting in the entry of a agent normally precluded from the mature CNS. Second, toxic substances that enter the CNS may differentially affect its various cell types. This is a result, in part, of biochemical differences in the cells, and regional variation in vascularization. Third, neurons once destroyed cannot be regenerated. As a result, cumulative losses of tissue or function can occur. Fourth, with respect to function, Norton (1978) points out that the nervous system possesses considerable reserve capacity. Structural redundancy is one source of reserve capacity and it may mask functional change until damage occurs in redundant structures. Finally, the nervous system often develops tolerance to a toxicant, resulting in the return of normal function despite the continuing presence of the toxicant.

3. Confounding Effects

Too often the occurrence of a broad spectrum of undesired or unexpected effects may confound the interpretation of behavioral changes associated with exposure to a toxicant. Such effects can include allergic reactions, idiosyncratic reactions, unexpected chemical interactions, immediate versus delayed toxicity, reversible versus irreversible toxic effects, and local versus systemic toxicity.

4. Behavioral Nonspecificity

A major problem associated with the use of behavioral tests is that is is often difficult to determine the specific contribution of sensory, motor, integrative, or emotional factors to a toxicant-related alteration in behavior. This lack of functional specificity can occur as a result of several factors. First, behavior is an integrative function, and, as such, reflects the status of many functional systems. Second, the majority of nervous system toxicants act at multiple sites and on multiple systems, and as a result, produce not one, but a broad range of functional disorders. Third, behavioral changes often occur as a result of indirect effects, such as toxicant-related changes at sites outside the nervous system. Weiss (1983) suggests several ways to manage these problems. First, neurobehavioral toxicologists should concentrate on identifying critical behavioral effects rather than broad or general changes. Specificity can be achieved through behavioral microanalysis and microcontrol strategies, and the use of sensitive instrumentation, multivariate-analysis procedures, and single-subject experimental designs.

5. Chronicity

Evans and Weiss (1978) used the term "chronicity factor" to emphasize the special importance of time course determinations in neurobehavioral toxicology and argue that neurobehavioral toxicologists must examine not only dose–effect relationships, but time–effect functions as well. Although many compounds enter and affect the CNS quite rapidly, a number of chemicals of interest to neurobehavioral toxicologists are characterized by slow uptake and elimination. These factors illustrate the need for threshold determinations and long-term behavioral studies. As these authors point out, continuous exposure to chemicals at doses below the threshold for observable acute effects may, given sufficient time, result in critical toxicant concentrations in target organs. Ultimately, the only constraint on exposure duration is the life span of the organism, and it is not clear that studies with short-lived animals can reveal the outcome of chronic exposure in long-lived animals. A subject which merits a considerable amount of study by neurobehavioral toxicologists is the interaction between toxicants and aging processes.

6. *Tolerance*

A well-known consequence of repeated administration of a chemical is the development of tolerance (Bignami *et al.*, 1975; Bignami, 1979). Most often tolerance refers to the observation that a reduction in any given effect of a chemical occurs when the same dose is administered repeatedly. Conversely, a larger dose is required to obtain the original effect. Tolerance has been observed in many situations using a number of different measurement techniques; therefore, it is not unexpected that several different forms of the phenomena have been described. Corfield-Sumner and Stolerman (1978) reviewed several forms of tolerance (behavioral, metabolic, learned, acute, cross, and reverse) and concluded that there is not adequate evidence to assume that tolerance to the behavioral effects of chemicals is essentially different from tolerance to their biochemical or physiological actions. Further, these authors observe that tolerance to the behavioral effects of a chemical is more likely to occur when a chemical is administered frequently, a range of dosages are employed, and exposure results in an initial loss of reinforcement or the suppression of a well-trained response. Given present knowledge, it is clear that a significant challenge for neurobehavioral toxicologists will be to assess the effect of tolerance phenomena on neurobehavioral toxicity.

IV. Corroborating Tests

As Evans and Weiss (1978) point out, too often behavioral toxicology studies are merely descriptive and do not address underlying mechanisms or provide the means for extrapolating findings to human beings. A frequent source of this problem is the absence of corroborating tests. Corroborating tests at the behavioral and nonbehavioral levels are necessary for a thorough understanding of the consequences of toxicant exposure.

At the behavioral level the simplest means of corroborating findings is test replication, or the use of a different test purporting to measure the same or similar function.

Although at the present level of technology functional changes can occur when no biochemical, morphological, or physiological changes are observable, the importance of nonbehavioral measures to understanding both functional change and overall neurotoxicity is clearly recognized (Merigan *et al.,* 1983; Norton, 1982; Damstra and Bondy, 1982; Fox *et al.,* 1982). Neurochemical studies can not only determine if a toxicant or its metabolites are present at target sites in the CNS, such studies can also aid in making inferences concerning mechanisms of action (Damstra and Bondy, 1982). Norton (1982) eloquently supports the need for morphological and chemical measures in assessing neurotoxicity by summarizing some basic principles for assessing organ damage: (1) all functional changes are the result of physical or chemical changes in cells; (2) organ damage can result in functional change; and (3) functional damage can be obscured by homeostatic mechanisms. Woolley (1977) discusses the value of electrophysiological tests in evaluating neurotoxicity and concludes that the principal advantages of such tests lie in their ability to assess the differential effects of a toxicant on distinct brain areas or systems, and in advancing the understanding of mechanisms of action. Recently published protocols for neurobehavioral toxicology research by the National Institute of Mental Health (NIMH, 1984) and the National Toxicology Program (NTP, 1984) specify that such studies include nonbehavioral measures. The neurobehavioral toxicology literature is replete with studies which employ nonbehavioral measures, and the use of these measures is becoming routine.

V. Neurobehavioral Assessment of Neurotoxins: Past and Present

A comprehensive review of the neurotoxins of past and current interest to neurobehavioral toxicologists is beyond the scope of the present chapter; therefore, the discussion that follows will be limited to an assessment of human exposure as a factor that has determined the neurotoxins investigators have chosen to study, and the identification of some of the neurotoxins that are at present actively being studied.

A. Human Exposure and the Study of Neurotoxins

As a developing research area neurobehavioral toxicology as yet lacks the direction of more established disciplines, and this is exemplified by the somewhat disparate group of neurotoxins that have, to date, been subjected to study. Further, of the neurotoxins studied, many have been subject to rigorous examination (lead, mercury), while others (solvents) have received only cursory study (NIMH, 1984). As previously mentioned, incidents of poisoning have perhaps been the single most influential factor in determining which neurotoxins have been studied. Classical examples are the 1929–1930 outbreak, in the United States, of "Jake-leg" paralysis resulting from tri-ortho-cresyl phosphate poisoning, the massive incident of methylmercury intoxication in Minamata and Niigata, Japan in the late 1950s, the more than 100 deaths which occurred in France in the 1950s as a result of organotin (diethyltin diiodide) exposure, and the more recent episodes in the United States of chlordecone poisoning in Hopewell, Virginia, Leptophos poisoning in Texas, and polybrominated biphenyl poisoning in Michigan (Schaumburg and Spender, 1980). Each of these neurotoxins has been extensively studied. In contrast, many neurotoxins have yet to be studied or require further evaluation, and an even greater number need to be examined under realistic conditions of exposure. Anger (1984) reported that of 588 chemicals for which standards were listed by the American Conference of Governmental Industrial Hygienists (ACGIH) in 1982, 167 had threshold limit values (TLVs) based on direct neurological or behavioral effects. More recently, Anger and Johnson (1985) identified several hundred neurotoxic chemicals from reference publications and found that of these only nine have been screened for neurobehavioral toxicity at existing industrial concentrations in workers. The tested chemicals included: carbon disulfide, carbon monoxide, formaldehyde, lead, mercury, methylchloride, perchloroethylene, polybrominated biphenyls, styrene, and trichloroethylene.

B. Neurotoxins of Current Interest

Although several alternatives for determining the chemicals that are of current interest to neurobehavioral toxicologists are available, short of a comprehensive review, two approaches seem useful. The first is to list the neurotoxins that have been the subject of recent symposia; the second is to list the neurotoxins employed in studies appearing in recent issues of key journals. Two periodicals, which in the judgment of the reviewer are considered key sources for the publication of neurobehavioral toxicology studies, were surveyed: *Neurotoxicology,* and *Neurobehavioral Toxicology and Teratology.* Presented in Table I is a list of symposia which were either announced or published in the 1983–1984 editions of these publications. The 11 symposia listed in Table I address more than a dozen chemicals. The majority of these agents are associated with incidences of exposure or chronic abuse problems. Presented in Table II is a list of the neurotoxins used in studies published in articles or abstracts in the 1984 issues of these journals. A total of 59 different neurotoxins were used in 198 studies. All of the chemicals listed are reported as having a neurotoxic effect. It is evident that a broad range of chemicals were studied including pesticides, metals, CNS drugs, therapeutic agents, food additives, solvents, gases, venoms, industrial pollutants, and many other types of chemicals. The data in Tables I and II reflect not only a healthy diversity of interests among neurobehavioral toxicologists, but also a significant interest in, and commitment to, neurobehavioral toxicology research.

VI. Topics for Future Research

Neurobehavioral toxicology will, in the future, continue to grow and become an increasingly important area of toxicology research. As more attention is focused on the behavioral effects of neurotoxins from within occupational medicine and from the public sector, interest in the behavioral effects of neurotoxins will grow, and demands for regulatory action will intensify. Indeed, regulatory agencies are presently experiencing such public concern (NPR, 1985). Given this, one of the major focuses of neurobehavioral toxicology research will be the continued development and validation of test procedures.

At present, one of the more active areas of neurobehavioral toxicology research concerns the functional consequences of the interaction of neurotoxins with developmental processes. In the past, the majority of toxicity testing was done in healthy adult male subjects. The importance of the prenatal and early postnatal periods was brought to the attention of neurobehavioral toxicologists by Pentschew and Garro (1966) and Spyker (1975a,b). This area of research has experienced tremendous growth in recent years and has become an autonomous area of endeavor (Snell, 1982; Yanai, 1984). Werboff and Gottlieb (1963) coined the term "behavioral teratology" to describe the area. Indeed, in a regulatory sense, behavioral teratology is ahead of

TABLE I

SYMPOSIA AND MEETINGS DIRECTED AT SPECIFIC NEUROTOXINS WHICH WERE ANNOUNCED OR PUBLISHED IN THE 1983–1984 VOLUMES OF *Neurotoxicology*, AND *Neurobehavioral Toxicology and Teratology*

Neurotoxin(s)	Symposium or meeting title
Ethanol	Fifth Annual Conference on Alcoholism entitled "Genetics and Alcoholism," held in El Paso, Texas, February 1981
Ethanol	First Congress of the International Society for Biomedical Research on Alcoholism, held in Munich, July 6–10, 1982
Lead	Lead Neurotoxicity Symposium, held in Chicago, September 20–21, 1982, as part of the First International Conference on Neurotoxicology of Selected Chemicals
Tin	Tin Neurotoxicity Symposium, held in Chicago, September 21–22, 1982, as part of the First International Conference on Neurotoxicology of Selected Chemicals
Manganese	First Manganese Neurotoxicity Symposium, held in Chicago, September 22–23, 1982, as part of the First International Conference on Neurotoxicology of Selected Chemicals
Metals (cadmium, lead, lithium, mercury)	"Recent Advances in Metal Toxicology," workshop held at Brookhaven National Laboratory, Upton, New York, October 11–12, 1982
Neurologic disease, chemically induced neurologic dysfunction	"Disease and Chemically Induced Neurological Dysfunction," workshop held in Raleigh, North Carolina, June 24–25, 1983
Ethanol	Kilian J. Schmitt Brain–Endocrine Interaction Symposium V, "Neuropeptides: Central and Peripheral," held in Würzburg, West Germany, July 27–29, 1983
Acrylamides, hexacarbons, IDPN, carbon disulfide	"Neurotoxicology of Selected Chemicals," symposium held in Chicago, September 11–15, 1983
Pyrethroids, other pesticides	Third International Conference on Neurotoxicology of Selected Chemicals, held in Chicago, September 9–12, 1984
Chemotherapeutic agents, over-the-counter drugs	"Neurotoxicology in the Fetus and Child," symposium held in Little Rock, Arkansas, September 9–13, 1985, as part of the Fourth International Conference on Neurotoxicology of Selected Chemicals

TABLE II

NEUROTOXINS INVESTIGATED IN ARTICLES AND ABSTRCTS IN THE 1984 VOLUMES OF *Neurotoxicology*, AND *Neurobehavioral Toxicology and Teratology*

Neurotoxin	Studies	Neurotoxin	Studies
Acrylamide	18	Lindane	3
Aflatoxin B_1	1	Lithium chloride	1
Aluminum chloride	1	Manganese	14
Amitraz	3	Methadone	3
Aspartame	1	Methyl *n*-butyl	1
β,β′-Iminodipropionitrile	1	Methylmercury	4
Bioresmethrin	1	*n*-Hexane	3
Cadmium	1	*n*-Propanol	1
Caffeine	1	Nicotine	1
Cannabis	1	*o,o,s*-Trimethylphosphorothiote	1
Carbon disulfide	2	Organophosphates	1
Carbon monoxide	1	*p*-Bromophenylacetylurea	3
Chloral	1	Paraoxon	2
Chlordecone	6	Permethrin	1
Chlordimeform	4	Phencyclidine	1
Cobalt	1	Physostigmine	1
Cyclodiene	1	Pralidoxime methanesulfonate	1
DDT	1	Pyrethroids	19
DFP	1	Sarin	1
Diazepam	2	Soman	1
Dichlorvos	1	Spider venom	1
Dieldrin	3	Tetrahydrocannabinol	1
Dithiobiuret	3	Tin	12
DMHD	1	Toluene	3
Doxorubicin	1	Triethyltin	1
Ethanol	11	Trimethylphosphate	1
Hexanedione	7	Trimethyltin	4
IDPN	10	Vasopressin	1
IDPN 2,6-heptanedione	1	Wasp venom	1
Kanamycin	1	Zine pyridinethione	1
Lead	23		

neurobehavioral toxicology in that Japan and Britain have regulations requiring that behavioral evaluations be done on all new drugs during premarket reproductive testing (Vorhees and Butcher, 1979). Vorhees (1983) outlines several lines of evidence which suggest that regulatory agencies in the United States may be giving regulation in this area serious consideration. In addition to the concern for the effects of neurotoxins on the developing nervous system, the aging brain is being recognized as an organ of special sensitivity (NIMH, 1984). The behavioral effects of neurotoxins may be exacerbated as a result of age-related loss of specific neuronal populations or the depletion of functional reserves associated with aging. The need for information regarding the behavioral effects of neurotoxins in the young and elderly is growing; therefore, these developmental periods will most probably be subject to extensive behavioral research.

Variables relating to the conditions of human exposure will be important topics for future neurobehavioral toxicology research. At present the majority of neurobehavioral toxicology studies concern the effects of a single chemical, whereas exposures most often occur to chemical mixtures. Similarly, behavioral studies are most frequently directed at healthy subjects; however, exposure occurs in organisms subjected to behavioral and physical stress (challenges). Although many organisms are exposed to neurotoxins over their life span, few studies address the neurobehavioral consequences of such long-term exposures. At present little is known about the mechanism of action of many neurotoxins, or how they may modify the synthesis, metabolism, and function of neurotransmitters or neuromodulators. Even less is known about the relationship of these changes to behavioral processes. The elucidation of these and many other issues awaits future study.

References

Anger, W. K. (1984). *Neurobehav. Toxicol. Teratol.* **6,** 147–153.

Anger, W. K., and Johnson, B. L. (1985). *In* "Neurotoxicity of Industrial and Commercial Chemicals" (J. L. O'Donoghue, ed.), Vol. 1, pp. 51–148. C.R.C. Press, Boca Raton, Florida.

Annau, Z. (1983). *In* "Application of Behavioral Pharmacology in Toxicology" (G. Zbinden, V. Cuomo, G. Racagni, and B. Weiss, eds.), pp. 87–95. Raven, New York.

Armstrong, R. D., Leach, L. J., Belluscio, P. R., Maynard, E. A., Hodge, H. C., and Scott, J. K. (1963). *Am. Ind. Hyg. Assoc. J.* **24,** 366–375.

Beard, R. R. (1974). *In* "Behavioral Toxicology: Early Detection of Occupational Hazards" (C. Xintaras, B. L. Johnson, and I. DeGroot, eds.), pp. 427–431. USGPO, Washington, D.C.

Beard, R. R., and Wertheim, G. A. (1967). *Am. J. Public Health* **57,** 2012–2022.

Bignami, G. (1976). *Annu. Rev. Pharmacol. Toxicol.* **16,** 329–366.

Bignami, G. (1979). *Neurobehav. Toxicol.* **1** (Suppl. 1), 179–186.

Bignami, G., Rosic, N., Michalek, H., Milosevic, M., and Gatti, G. L. (1975). *In* "Behavioral Toxicology" (B. Weiss and V. Laties, eds.), pp. 155–210. Plenum, New York.

Brimblecombe, R. W. (1968). *In* "Modern Trends in Toxicology" (E. Boyland and R. Goulding, eds.), pp. 149–174. Butterworths, London.

Brimblecombe, R. W. (1976). *Clin. Toxicol.* **9,** 731–743.

Butcher, R. E. (1976). *Environ. Health Perspect.* **18,** 75–78.

Cabe, P. A., and Eckerman, D. A. (1982). *In* "Nervous System Toxicology" (C. L. Mitchell, ed.), pp. 133–198. Raven, New York.

Casarett, L. J. (1975). *In* "Toxicology The Basic Science of Poisons" (L. J. Casarett and J. Doull, eds.), pp. 3–10. Macmillan, New York.

Corfield-Sumner, P. K., and Stolerman, I. P. (1978). *In* "Contemporary Research in Behavioral Pharmacology" (D. E. Blackman and D. J. Sanger, eds.), pp. 391–448. Plenum, New York.

Damstra, T., and Bondy, S. C. (1982). *In* "Nervous System Toxicology" (C. L. Mitchell, ed.), pp. 349–373. Raven, New York.

Davis, J. M. (1982). *In* "Nervous System Toxicology" (C. L. Mitchell, ed.), pp. 29–44. Raven, New York.

Dews, P. D., and Wenger, G. R. (1979). *Neurobehav. Toxicol.* **1** (Suppl. 1), 119–127.

Donovick, P. J., and Horowitz, G. P. (1982). *J. Toxicol. Environ. Health* **10,** 1–9.

Evans, H. L., and Weiss, B. (1978). *In* "Contemporary Research in Behavioral Pharmacology" (D. E. Blackman and D. J. Sanger, eds.), pp. 449–487. Plenum, New York.

Fox, D. A., Lowndes, H. E., and Bierkamper, G. G. (1982). *In* "Nervous System Toxicology" (C. L. Mitchell, ed.), pp. 299–335. Raven, New York.

Gad, S. C. (1981). *Toxicologist* **1,** 150.

Gehring, P. J., and Rao, K. S. (1979). *In* "Patty's Industrial Hygiene and Toxicology" (L. J. Cralley and L. V. Cralley, eds.), Vol. 3, pp. 567–594. Wiley, New York.

Geller, I., Stebbins, W. C., and Wayner, M. J., eds. (1979). *Neurobehav. Toxicol.* **1** (Suppl. 1).

Goldberg, M. E., Haun, C., and Smyth, H. F. (1962). *Toxicol. Appl. Pharmacol.* **4,** 148–164.

Hopper, D. L. (1985). *In* "Safety Evaluation of Drugs and Chemicals" (W. E. Lloyd ed.), Hemisphere Publ., Washington, D.C. (in press).

Hopper, D. L. (1986). *In* "Safety Evaluation of Drugs and Chemicals" (W. E. Lloyd, ed.), pp. 305–321. Hemisphere, Washington, D.C.

Mello, N. K. (1975). *Fed. Proc., Fed. Am. Soc. Exp. Biol.* **34,** 1832–1834.

Merigan, W. H., Maurissen, J. P., Barkdoll, E., Eskin, T. A., and Lapham, L. W. (1983). *In* "Application of Behavioral Pharmacology in Toxicology" (G. Zbinden, V. Cuomo, G. Racagni, and B. Weiss, eds.), pp. 113–126. Raven, New York.

Mitchell, C. L. (1978). *Environ. Health Perspect.* **26,** 3–4.

Mitchell, C. L., ed. (1982). "Nervous System Toxicology." Raven, New York.

Mitchell, C. L., and Tilson, H. A. (1982). *CRC Crit. Rev. Toxicol.* **10,** 265–274.

Mitchell, C. L., Tilson, H. A., and Cabe, P. A. (1982). *In* "Nervous System Toxicology" (C. L. Mitchell, ed.), pp. 237–245. Raven, New York.

Morgan, B. B., and Repko, J. (1974). *In* "Behavioral Toxicology: Early Detection of Occupational Hazards" (C. Xintaras, B. L. Johnson, and I. DeGroot, eds.), pp. 478–479. USGPO, Washington, D.C.

Munsch, M. H., and Potter, R. L. (1979). *In* "Patty's Industrial Hygiene and Toxicology" (L. J. Cralley and L. V. Cralley, eds.), Vol. 3, pp. 681–718. Wiley, New York.

NAS (1975). "Principles for Evaluating Chemicals in the Environment." National Academy of Sciences, Washington, D.C.

NAS (1977). "Principles and Procedures for Evaluating the Toxicity of Household Substances." National Academy of Sciences, Washington, D.C.

NIMH (1984). "The Neuroscience of Mental Health." National Institute of Mental Health, Rockville, Maryland.

Norton, S. (1978). *Environ. Health Perspect.* **26,** 21–27.

Norton, S. (1980). *In* "Toxicology The Basic Science of Poisons" (L. J. Casarett and J. Boull, eds.), pp. 179–205. Macmillan, New York.

Norton, S. (1982). *In* "Principles and Methods of Toxicology" (A. W. Hayes, ed), pp. 353–373. Raven, New York.

NPR (1985). "Chemicals in the Workplace" (D. Zwerdling, ed.). National Public Radio, Washington, D.C.

NRC/NAS (1984). "Toxicity Testing: Strategies to Determine Needs and Priorities." National Academy Press, Washington, D.C.

NTP (1984). "National Toxicology Program, Fiscal Year 1984 Annual Plan." U.S. Department of Health and Human Services.

Nunnally, J. C. (1967). "Psychometric Theory." McGraw-Hill, New York.

Page, N. P. (1979). *Neurobeh. Toxicol.* **1** (Suppl. 1), 3–5.

Pavlenko, S. M. (1975). *In* "Methods Used in the USSR for Establishing Biologically Safe Levels of Toxic Substances," pp. 86–108. World Health Organization, Geneva.

Pentschew, A., and Garro, F. (1966). *Acta Neuropathol.* **6,** 266–278.

Reiter, L. (1978). *Environ. Health Perspect.* **26,** 5–7.

Reiter, L. W. (1980). *Neurobeh. Toxicol.* **2,** 73–74.

Reiter, L. W., MacPhail, R. C., Fuppert, P. H., and Eckerman, D. A. (1981). *Proc. Conf. Environ. Toxicol., 11th,* **11,** 11–23.

Ruffin, J. B. (1963). *J. Occup. Med.* **5,** 117.

Russell, R. W., and Singer, G. (1982). *Neurobehav. Toxicol. Teratol.* **4,** 5–7.

Sandler, B., Van Gelder, G. A., Buck, W. B., Maland, J. B., and Karas, G. G. (1968). *Psychol. Rep.* **23,** 451–455.

Sandler, B., Van Gelder, G. A. Elsberry, D. Dk., and Karas, G. G. (1969). *Psychon. Sci.* **15,** 261.

Silverman, P. (1974). *New Sci.* **67,** 255–258.

Snell, K., ed. (1982). "Developmental Toxicology." Croom-Helm, London.

Spencer, P. S., and Schaumburg, H. H., eds. (1980). "Experimental and Clinical Neurotoxicology." Williams & Wilkins, Baltimore.

Spyker, J. M. (1974). *In* "Behavioral Toxicology: Early Detection of Occupational Hazards" (C. Xintaras, B. L. Johnson, and I. DeGroot, eds.), pp. 470–477. USGPO, Washington, D.C.

Spyker, J. M. (1975a). *In* "Behavioral Toxicology" (B. Weiss and V. G. Laties, eds.), pp. 311–344. Plenum, New York.

Spyker, J. M. (1975b). *Fed. Proc., Fed. Am. Soc. Exp. Biol.* **34,** 1835–1844.

Spyker, J. M., and Goad, P. T. (1983). *In* "Application of Behavioral Pharmacology in Toxicology" (G. Zbinden, V. Cuomo, G. Bacagni, and B. Weiss, eds.), pp. 97–112. Raven, New York.

Stebbins, W. C. (1982). *Environ. Health Perspect.* **44,** 77–85.

Thompson, T., and Schuster, C. R. (1968). "Behavioral Pharamacology." Prentice-Hall, New York.

Tilson, H. A., and Cabe, P. A. (1978). *Environ. Health Perspect.* **26,** 287–299.

Tilson, H. A., and Harry, G. J. (1982). *In* "Nervous System Toxicology" (C. L. Mitchell, ed.), pp. 1–27. Raven, New York.

Tilson, H. A., and Mitchell, C. L. (1984). *Annu. Rev. Pharmacol. Toxicol.* **24,** 425–450.

Tilson, H. A., Mitchell, C. L., and Cabe, P. A. (1979). *Neurobehav. Toxicol.* **1** (Suppl. 1), 137–148.

Tilson, H. A., Cabe, P. A., and Burne, T. A. (1980). *In* "Experimental and Clinical Neurotoxicology" (P. S. Spencer and H. H. Schaumburg, eds.). Williams & Wilkins, Baltimore.

Van Gelder, G. A., and Smith, R. M. (1973). *Toxicol. Appl. Pharmacol.* **25,** 485.

Van Gelder, G. A., Buck, W. B., and Karas, G. G. (1968). *Ind. Med. Surg.* **37,** 528.

Van Gelder, G. A., Buck, W. B., and Karas, G. G. (1970). *J. Am. Vet. Med. Assoc.* **156,** 1208.

Van Gelder, G. A., Carson, T. L., and Buck, W. B. (1973). *Toxicol. Appl. Pharmacol.* **25,** 466.

Vorhees, C. V. (1983). *Neurobehav. Toxicol. Teratol.* **5,** 469–474.

Vorhees, C. V., and Butcher, R. R. (1979). *In* "Developmental Toxicology" (K. Snell, ed.), pp. 247–298. Croom-Helm, London.

Weiss, B. (1983). *In* "Application of Behavioral Pharmacology in Toxicology" (G. Zbinden, V. Cuomo, G. Racagni, and B. Weiss, eds.), pp. 71–86. Raven, New York.

Weiss, B., and Laties, V. (1969). *Annu. Rev. Pharmacol.* **9,** 297–326.

Weiss, B., and Laties, V. G., eds. (1975). "Behavioral Toxicology." Plenum, New York.

Weiss, B., and Laties, V. G. (1979). *Neurobehav. Toxicol.* **1** (Suppl. 1), 213–215.

Werboff, J., and Gottlieb, J. S. (1963). *Obstet. Gynecol. Surv.* **18,** 420–423.

Woolley, D. E. (1977). *In* "Behavioral Toxicology: An Emerging Discipline," pp. 9(1)–9(25). U.S. Environmental Protection Agency, Research Triangle Park, North Carolina.

Xintaras, C., and Burg, J. R. (1980). *In* "Experimental and Clinical Neurotoxicology" (P. S. Spencer and H. H. Schaumburg, eds.), pp. 663–674. Williams & Wilkins, Baltimore.

Xintaras, C., and Johnson, B. L. (1976). *In* "Essays in Toxicology" (W. J. Hayes, ed.), Vol. 7, pp. 155–201. Academic Press, New York.

Xintaras, C., Johnson, B. L., and DeGroot, I., eds. (1974). "Behavioral Toxicology: Early Detection of Occupational Hazards." USGPO, Washington, D.C.

Yanai, J., ed. (1984). "Neurobehavioral Teratology." Elsevier, New York.

Zbinden, G. (1983). *In* "Application of Behavioral Pharmacology in Toxicology" (G. Zbinden, V. Cuomo, G. Racagni, and B. Weiss, eds.), pp. 1–14. Raven, New York.

Zbinden, G., Cuomo, V., Racagni, G., and Weiss, B., eds. (1983). "Application of Behavioral Pharmacology in Toxicology." Raven, New York.

Zenick, H., and Reiter, L. W., eds. (1977). "Behavioral Toxicology: An Emerging Discipline." U.S. Environmental Protection Agency, Research Triangle Park, North Carolina.

Immunotoxicology

G. DESCOTES* AND G. MAZUÉ†

*Centre de Recherches Clin-Midy/Sanofi, F-34082 Montpellier, France

†Farmitalia Carlo Erba, Viale E. Bezzi, I-20146 Milan, Italy

I. Introduction

Toxicology is a rapidly changing field. Once an essentially descriptive science, it has become investigative, attempting to elucidate mechanisms responsible for the toxic effects observed. The toxicologist is aided in this work by specialists in ophthalmology, hematology, biochemistry, and immunology. The purpose of toxicity studies is to investigate or confirm side effects of a foreign compound in laboratory animals and, when possible from the information gathered, to assess the impact of the compound in the species for which it is intended. For this, two approaches are used by the toxicologist: (1) routine toxicity testing (acute, chronic toxicity, etc.) and (2) studies specifically designed to explore particular systems, such as the immune system.

Over the past few years a number of articles on immunotoxicology have been published. Professional organizations, scientific societies, and regulatory authorities at the national and international levels have all organized seminars around this theme. Is immunotoxicology a necessity or merely a fashionable trend? What is its role in modern toxicology?

The immune system, like the other systems which together make up an organism (animal or plant), has many functions and therefore must also be closely evaluated during toxicity studies in vertebrates. Its classical role is the protection of the organism against external aggression; however, the response can be excessive (hypersensitivity or allergy) or insufficient (increased susceptibility to infections). The immune system also aids in maintaining homeostasis; the loss of this equilibrium leads to autoimmune diseases. Finally it regulates and destroys aberrant cells, such as tumor cells; loss of this control system can result in cancer.

II. Brief Anatomical and Physiological Considerations

The immune system, though organized according to a strict hierarchy, remains dynamic to cope with its variety of functions. Precursors of immune system cells derive from bone marrow stem cells. Of these, the lymphocytes mature in central lymphoid tissues such as the thymus (for future T cells) and the bursa of Fabricius or bone marrow (for future B cells); they then travel to peripheral lymphoid tissues such as the spleen and the lymph nodes, or diffuse tissues such as the gut-associated lymphoid tissue (GALT) and others which provide mucosal-associated immunity. Some of these cells differentiate on antigenic stimulation and become the elements of the specific immune response. Other cells of the immune system (mononuclear phagocytes and polymorphonuclear leukocytes) are capable of maturing outside of the central lymphoid tissues.

A. Central Lymphoid Tissues

Central lymphoid tissues appear at an early stage during embryonic tissue development. They provide a protective and inductive environment for the stem cells that colonize them. They are the site of intense lymphocyte proliferation which is independent of any antigenic stimulation and which needs only a constant supply of bone marrow lymphoid stem cells. The thymus is the best example of this (and is the only macroscopically identifiable lymphoid organ in mammals); in this organ of lymphoepithelial structure, the future T cells proliferate, differentiate, and mature in contact with the epithelium, aided by thymic factors secreted by the epithelial cells. These young T cells migrate via the bloodstream to thymodependent areas of peripheral lymphoid tissues and, having become differentiated T cells, they will never return to the thymus. In birds and reptiles, the bursa of Fabricius is to B lymphocytes what the thymus is to T lymphocytes, whereas in mammals the bone marrow is probably the site of B lymphocyte maturation.

B. Peripheral Lymphoid Tissues

Peripheral lymphoid tissues are effectors of the immune system. They only develop naturally under antigenic stimulation and are found on the entry routes of antigens: spleen for systemic contact, lymph nodes of the cutaneous tissues for dermal aggression, tonsils and lymph nodes of the respiratory tract for airborne xenobiotics, and lymph nodes of the gastrointestinal tract for food contacts. The major production of antibodies and sensitized cells takes place here, and thus, these tissues undergo constant change. The general organization of peripheral lymphoid tissues is that of a conjunctive structure accommodating the different protagonists of the immune response: macrophages that entrap the antigen and small masses of lymphocytes that give rise to sensitized cells and antibody-producing cells. The structures of the splenic white pulp and the lymph nodes are homologous: a B-type follicular zone (peripheral regions of the white pulp and cortical area of the lymph nodes), a T-type zone (periarteriolar regions of the white pulp and paracortical area of the lymph nodes), and finally a medullary zone rich in macrophages and plasmocytes. Numerous other lymphoid formations are spread throughout the body, mainly along the length of the respiratory and digestive tracts. Tonsils and Peyer's patches are lymphoid islets with a general organization less complex than that of the previously cited large peripheral tissues; they are above all rich in IgA-producing cells and play an essential role in mucosal-associated immunity.

C. Cells of the Immune Response

All the cells of the immune system are derived from pluripotent stem cells of the bone marrow and undergo differentiation. Mononuclear phagocytes and polynucleated leukocytes do not need passage through central lymphoid organs to acquire their specific characteristics, whereas lymphocytes do.

The mononuclear phagocytes act as inductors of an immune response by presenting the antigen to the T lymphocytes and by producing a variety of monokines such as interleukin 1 (IL-1), previously named lymphocyte-activating factor. They are also the effectors of some specific immune responses using the Fc and C3b receptors on their membrane; these receptors facilitate specifically the phagocytosis of exogenous particles, which is one of the simplest defense mechanisms. Macrophages immobilize, then neutralize the particle, thus playing an important role against microbial invasion (specific immune response intervenes afterwards). These cells may also play a role in immune surveillance of tumor growth by directly lysing tumor cells. Polymorphonuclear neutrophils also neutralize exogenous microorganisms and carry membrane receptors for the Fc fragment of IgG and for C3b. Thus, they act as effectors of immune response, but since they are unable to transfer antigen information to lymphocytes, they cannot act as inductors. The other polynucleated leukocytes, eosinophils and basophils, as well as their equivalents in tissues (mastocytes), are effectors in allergy-type immune responses.

T and B lymphocytes are involved in the specific immune response. In brief, after the presentation by the macrophages of the foreign antigen in association with major histocompatibility complex products, lymphocytes express receptors to IL-1 and begin to produce interleukin 2 (IL-2), previously named T-cell growth factor, which induces proliferation of other T cells (including helper T cells which produce IL-2 themselves). These T cells multiply and differentiate into several subpopulations (amplifier, memory, and suppressor T cells) and act on B lymphocytes that become plasmocytes, specific antibody producers. In parallel, other sensitized T lymphocytes can differentiate into effectors of non-antibody-mediated specific immunity (called cell-mediated immunity): effectors of delayed-type hypersensitivity and of allograft rejection, effectors of the graft versus host reaction, and cytotoxic T lymphocytes. At different stages of this cascade, soluble mediators (interleukins and interferons) regulate cooperation between the cells. Apart from these well-documented cell types, there are other cells which are better defined by their activity than by their morphology or their surface markers: the natural killer (NK) cells and the large granular lymphocytes of the gut. Both are capable of spontaneously killing tumor cells and are suspected of being involved in tumor surveillance. The killer (K) cells responsible for the antibody-dependent cellular cytotoxicity response could be classed here because the majority of them also exhibit NK activity.

D. Applications

In conclusion, the effect of a foreign substance on the immune system can be assessed by (1) the quantification of the system's components during toxicity studies (routine hematology and histological examination of controls and treated animals), (2) the *in vitro* examination of the capabilities of the immune system components, and (3) the comparison of overall immune response of compound-treated animals with that of placebo-treated controls. Various methods could be used to evaluate these immune responses: natural resistance to a pathogenic microbe, specific humoral or cellular immune response to an antigen, and even immune response against the compound itself (i.e., allergy).

III. Proposed Models for Immunotoxicity Assessment

A. General Considerations

Tests for evaluating compound immunotoxicity are very different according to whether they are proposed by an immunologist or by a toxicologist, except for animal models routinely used to evaluate allergenic potential of drugs or chemicals. An immunologist would choose classical immunopharmacological tests, usually carried out in small laboratory animals, to detect any immunomodulating properties (including immunotoxic side effects) of a test compound. A toxicologist would use routine animal toxicity studies giving an abundance of information that is, however, of a static nature (e.g., white cell count and microscopic examination of the spleen) and shed little light on the functional capacities of the immune system. Nevertheless, a well-carried-out toxicity study rarely fails to detect a serious problem and alerts the toxicologist to the possibility of immune system defects: signs of microbial infection or allergic reactions to the compound will be noted during clinical examination and necropsy. Therefore, modern toxicology should be based on cooperation between different disciplines, including immunology, just as an efficient immune response is based on a harmonious cooperation between different elements of the immune system.

In the late 1970s, several pioneers in immunotoxicology attempted to use classical models of immunopharmacology for work in this field (Vos, 1977; Dean *et al.*, 1979a; Luster and Faith, 1979). This was followed by a host of publications putting forward numerous test models yielding results sometimes difficult to extrapolate to the species for which the products were intended: human beings, farm animals, and pets. In the light of these developments, limits to the use of these models were drawn up, as defined by one team (Dean *et al.*, 1983):

> The selection and validation of these immunological methods for toxicological studies have addressed several issues. These include the following: (1) does the method yield results that are consistent and reproducible within and between

> laboratories?; (2) does the method have sufficient sensitivity to detect biologically significant changes (e.g., alterations in host susceptibility to infectious agents or neoplastic cell growth?; (3) does the method predict immunotoxic potential in humans?

Two further questions should be added today to this list: (1) Are all these tests necessary? and (2) does the quality of the information justify their cost? Other disciplines have likewise undergone difficult beginnings before becoming established. After a dramatic increase in the number of tests proposed for evaluating compound mutagenicity, currently only a few are in routine use because of their predictive value and low cost. In the near future, perhaps only three or four routine, inexpensive, and reliable tests will suffice to assess immunotoxic potential.

Briefly, immunotoxicological tests can be grouped according to (1) the type of approach (overall or specific) or (2) the type of immunity evaluated (nonspecific, humoral, cellular, or antitumoral) or drug allergy. Some of these tests have been validated using known immunotoxic compounds in humans and/or animals, and most have already been described in detail elsewhere. Screening tests for classical immunotoxicity evaluation are proposed in Table I. Points to consider in their selection and in in-depth testing are discussed below.

B. Protocol Conditions

1. Species

Routine toxicity studies are performed in outbred dogs, monkeys, rabbits, and rats, but rarely in mice except for carcinogenicity tests carried out on hybrid mice (e.g., B6C3F1). Immunopharmacological tests applied to toxicology are performed in the mouse because of its well-known immune system. Since outbred mice are inexpensive, they should be used whenever possible. However, inbred mice are necessary whenever a histocompatibility barrier is required (such as for syngeneic tumor challenge or allograft rejection); these tests are therefore more costly, and their results are sometimes more difficult to extrapolate because of murine strain-specific differences in enzyme activity (e.g., Vecchi *et al.*, 1983). The guinea pig is used to evaluate allergenic potential of a compound because of its particular sensitivity. In addition, the animals' state of health should also be taken into account; for example, during toxicity studies of immunosuppressive agents, latent pathological infection could be manifest in captured animals such as monkeys, whereas this effect would not appear in specific pathogen-

TABLE I

ANIMAL MODELS PROPOSED FOR PRIMARY IMMUNOTOXICITY EVALUATION[a]

Type of immunity	Tests	Alternative techniques
Nonspecific	Resistance to *Listeria monocytogenes*	Resistance to *Klebsiella pneumoniae* or *Streptococcus pneumoniae*
	Lewis lung carcinoma challenge	B16F10 or PYB6 tumor challenge
Humoral	Primary antibody response to T-dependent antigen: PFC technique	Same approach using direct hemagglutination or hemolysis technique
	Antibody response to T-independent antigen: LPS	Same approach using SSS-III
Cell mediated	Footpad assay	Oxazolone sensitization
	Tumor allograft rejection[b]: L1210	Same approach using other tumors routinely maintained in the laboratory
Hypersensitivity	Open epicutaneous test (for contact allergens)	Magnusson and Kligman's test
	Photoallergenicity testing (for photo-unstable compounds)	

[a]No further testing required in the absence of modifications.
[b]Performed only in the event of modification detected in the preceding test in the list.

free rats raised under hygienic conditions. Moreover, animals used for the examination of a particular immune response could provide false results if their responses are already altered by infection (Boorman *et al.*, 1982).

2. *Compound Administration*

For *in vivo* or *ex vivo* studies, the drug is administered by the route that induces immune disturbances in toxicity studies or intended for use in human beings (e.g., oral administration for food additives or topical administration for cosmetic creams), and using the same solvent or vehicle (a control group will receive the same volume of solvent alone). For *in vitro* studies, particular attention should be paid to the solubility of the compound and osmolarity and pH of the medium; adequate controls should therefore be carried out. Furthermore, test repeatability can only be guaranteed if certain factors are checked beforehand (e.g., spontaneous mitogenic activity or enzyme activity of fetal calf serum).

3. Dose Range Finding

Normally, at least three dose levels are used, generally four, geometrically spread from the therapeutic dose level to a dose level that provokes toxic effects (causing at least a 10% decrease in body weight). While this approach is valid in the case of direct toxicity (e.g., myelotoxicity), it is not in the case of drug-related allergy because the optimum response may occur at dose levels below the upper limit of the range.

4. Duration of Chemical Exposure

Duration of chemical exposure depends on the intended use or the drug family. An antibiotic is prescribed for a short period of time in humans or domestic animals; therefore, a short experimental treatment period (1–2 weeks) is sufficient for the evaluation of potential immunosuppressive side effects (but gives no indication of possible allergenic effects). Conversely, for a drug that is taken over a longer time (minor tranquilizers, antiarrhythmic agents), animals should be treated daily for a longer period (i.e., 1 month). In screening studies, an immune response (i.e., first contact with antigen, followed by specific response, and finally, possible second contact with the antigen) should be elicited during the treatment of the animals with the test compound and, in the event of immune alteration, follow-up studies will pinpoint the most sensitive period of chemical exposure. In experimental infections the infective bolus is administered, for practical reasons, on the last day of compound treatment. For the detection of drug-induced allergies, treatment is split into several periods (sensitization, rest, challenge). These protocols are described in Section III,F.

5. Chemical Exposure Conditions

The first-step tests should be performed *in vivo* because they are more realistic: they take into account compound absorption, metabolism, and possible direct toxicity to other organs (hepatotoxicity can be accompanied by humoral deficiency owing to inhibited protein synthesis). Most of these tests can be performed without sophisticated equipment, validated using positive controls, and conducted by any toxicology laboratory. *In vitro* tests often require expensive equipment (CO_2 incubator, laminar-flow hood, β and/or γ counters, and radiolabeled compounds subject to safety regulations). Furthermore, results obtained *in vitro* must be correlated with effects observed *in vivo,* because cells in culture are more susceptible to damage in the nonphysiological and relatively dilute microenvironment. Once the predictive value of the *in vitro* tests is well established, they will present obvious advantages as alternative tests.

C. Nonspecific Immunity

The division between nonspecific and specific immunity is essentially for descriptive purposes, because the immune process is a continuum in which the specific immunity follows rapidly the nonspecific events to ensure complete protection of the organism. The major cells involved in nonspecific immunity are the mononucleated cells: blood monocytes and histiocytes of the tissues (as diverse as the alveolar macrophages of the lung, resident peritoneal macrophages, Kupffer cells of the liver, microglial cells of the central nervous system, and Langerhans cells of the skin); polynuclear neutrophils, and K and NK cells are involved to a lesser extent. Mononuclear cells also play a key role in specific humoral and cellular immunity; any alteration in their function induces either positive or negative immune modifications. Increasing host resistance by pharmacological activation of these cells is a major goal of immunopharmacology.

Examples of congenital or acquired immune alterations exist in human beings, illustrating the importance of assessing nonspecific immunity. Patients who receive prolonged immunosuppressive therapy to prevent graft rejection are more susceptible to infection, especially with opportunistic organisms, and have a higher incidence of tumors than normal populations (Penn, 1978). In the same way, laboratory animals treated with immunosuppressive compounds show greater susceptibility to experimental infections, transplantable tumors, and sometimes spontaneous tumors. Resistance to experimental infection and/or rejection of syngeneic tumors are thus logical models to detect compounds with immunotoxic side effects.

As a first-step model, we test natural resistance to *Listeria monocytogenes*. In the normal host, the destruction of this facultative intracellular bacterium requires (1) immediate phagocytosis and killing by mononucleated cells and (2) specific cellular immune response mediated by T cells (more than 2 days after the inoculation) (Tripathy and Mackaness, 1969). The exact quantity of bacteria needed depends on age, weight, sex, etc., of recipients and thus can be difficult to determine precisely. For this reason, two experiments are run in parallel, one with an amount of bacteria likely to kill 0–20% of controls and the other amount likely to kill 60–80% of controls; either positive (protective) or negative effect of the test compound, therefore, would be detected. The routes for treatment and for infection should be different because of the possibility of only a local disturbance of the mononuclear cells (e.g., peritoneal macrophages). Changes in the host defense to *Listeria* infection are most easily assessed by calculating total mortality rate and mean survival time. On the finding of greater susceptibility, bacterial colony counts from liver and spleen (major sites for replication) at different postinfection days give additional information on the precise cellular target of the immune system: differences in counts are correlated the second day following infection with macrophage activity, and after the fourth or fifth day with T-cell activity.

The *Listeria* infection model appears to be the most frequently used; however, other bacteria have been proposed. *Klebsiella pneumoniae* infection is a well-known model, which we find less practical because the mice die too quickly and specific humoral immunity has little time to intervene. This test is rather used to select biological response modifiers which activate macrophages. The *Streptococcus pneumoniae* infection model is worth noting. T-Independent antibodies to the pneumococcal polysaccharides represent the second line of defense against this bacterium (Winkelstein and Swift, 1975) and are opsonizing antibodies which markedly enhance phagocytic capacity of mononucleated cells and polymorphonuclear leukocytes. Thus this model could be eventually developed for evaluating this particular aspect. Fungi (*Candida albicans*), parasites (*Trichinella spiralis*), and viruses (herpes simplex virus, cytomegalovirus) can also be used. The *Candida* infection model has an advantage in that it reveals in particular polymorphonuclear leukocyte damage (Hurtrel *et al.,* 1980), severity of which could be determined by calculating total mortality rate and/or by counting the colonies under the renal capsule or by plating the homogenized kidneys. *Trichinella spiralis* expulsion is a model in which T-cell immunity plays a major role (Larsh *et al.,* 1974) and is used by several groups of investigators. The major viral models, with their advantages and disadvantages, are described in detail by Kern (1982). During viral infections, the organism's defense involves first an early interferon response (Gresser *et al.,* 1976), then cooperation between mononucleated cells, NK cells, helper and cytotoxic T cells, and also B cells producing neutralizing antibodies. In summary, even though there are some similarities in the mechanisms of resistance to different microbial infections, there are also differences, as shown by varying degrees of susceptibility induced by the same drug (Morahan *et al.*, 1979). Therefore, more than one test should be used for compound screening. In the event of altered resistance, additional tests can identify the compound effects on target cells or their functions.

NK cells, macrophages, and lymphocytes play also a major role in the "immune surveillance" of tumors (Burnet, 1970), and immunosuppressive drugs increase the incidence of cancer by acting on them. Thus, a drug's impact has to be evaluated on the organism's capacity to (1) reject grafted syngeneic tumor and (2) prevent development of spontaneous tumors. The latter aspect is well covered during carcinogenicity studies, but a long observation period is required. Various models are proposed to evaluate the former. One routinely used model is the challenge of treated syngeneic mice by intravenous injection of a suspension of dissociated Lewis lung carcinoma cells to induce small tumor masses as for experimental pulmonary metastasis. After approximately 20 days, the pulmonary tumors are counted and their diameter measured. (The exact autopsy date will depend on the sensitivity of the mice because under immunosuppressive drug regimens, the tumor kills the mice earlier and necessitates an earlier autopsy.) Other tumors, such as the B16F10 melanoma, which have a high lung colonization potential, can also be used. Even better tumor cell concentration per organ can be precisely determined by the use of radioactive markers such as ^{125}[I]iododeoxyuridine, but the problem of radioactive waste is encountered. Other tests use death as an end point: syngeneic mice are injected with one of the numerous murine tumors routinely maintained in immunology laboratories, and death due to tumor is daily recorded. One such system using the PYB6 sarcoma has been described by Dean *et al.* (1979b).

Any alteration of resistance to infection or to syngeneic tumor challenge alerts the investigator to the necessity for further exploratory tests. For example, because NK cells play a key role in tumor surveillance (Hanna and Burton, 1981; reviewed by Herberman, 1982), NK activity should be evaluated in the case of tumor rejection defect. This is done *in vitro* and/or *ex vivo* using target cells labeled with ^{51}Cr according to Mantovani *et al.* (1978) (YAC-1 cells for mouse NK activity and K562 cells for rat or monkey NK activity). In the *in vivo* method, YAC-1 cells labeled with ^{125}[I]iododeoxyuridine are directly injected into mice, and the organ NK activity is correlated with its radioactivity level (Riccardi *et al.*, 1979).

In summary, numerous tests for evaluating nonspecific immunity are available, both *in vivo* and *in vitro*. We must take into account in selecting *in vitro* tests that the assessment of the functions of the cells responsible for the first line of defense is complicated because of (1) the vast number of assays available, (2) the multiple functions of these cells, (3) the various sources from which they can be harvested, and (4) the different stages at which they are obtained (resident, inflammatory, cytotoxic, activated, etc.). Also, some of these occasionally give information in apparent contradiction with general effects observed *in vivo*. For example, diethylstilbestrol increases some macrophage functions (Boorman *et al.*, 1980), while it decreases resistance to *L. monocytogenes* and to syngeneic tumor challenges (Dean *et al.*, 1980). The tumor promoter phorbol myristate acetate inhibits *in vitro* the cytolytic capacity of activated macrophages (Keller, 1979; Fish *et al.*, 1981), whereas it enhances the resistance to *Listeria* but decreases syngeneic tumor rejection capacity (Murray *et al.*, 1985).

These examples show the discrepancy between *in vitro* and *in vivo* tests. The *in vivo* tests should be preferred to *in vitro* ones, which only examine one function of cells from one source, at one stage. These examples also show the necessity of undertaking more than one *in vivo* test to evaluate the real compound impact on nonspecific immunity.

D. Humoral Immunity

During routine toxicity studies, signs of possible disturbance in humoral immunity would be noted by determination of serum total protein and globulin, by clinical observation of possible gastrointestinal or respiratory pathology, and by histological examination of lymphoid organs.

A specific approach to evaluate humoral immunity, which is also simple, direct, inexpensive, and safe for the worker is to measure the antibody response of small animal species after immunization with a thymodependent antigen, the most commonly encountered. The most often used antigen is sheep red blood cells (SRBC), and in this case, the primary immune response (IgM) is evaluated by direct measurement of the target cell lysis in the presence of complement [and the secondary response (IgG) when specific anti-IgG serum is added]. The most well-known method is the enumeration of splenocytes capable of releasing lytic antibodies to red cells which are plated around them (plaque-forming cells, PFC) in solid medium, as first described by Jerne and Nordin (1963), or in liquid medium (Cunningham and Szenberg, 1968). The PFC technique (direct for IgM or indirect for IgG) has the advantage of providing a measurement of the spleen cellularity as well as an opportunity to examine other lymphoid tissues of the killed animals (e.g., the thymus). However, the same animal cannot be used for measuring both primary and secondary responses at different intervals. This is possible if the circulating antibodies are evaluated by the second best known methods: direct hemagglutination or hemolysis in microplates. The advantages of these methods are that (1) a very small quantity of serum is required and, because animals are not killed, they can receive a booster injection while being treated with the compound, and that (2) as sera can be frozen, several assays can be performed on the same day, saving time and money. Whereas the PFC method measures antibody-release cell capacity, the second methods only measure the circulating antibodies at a given moment. Although our own experience shows good correlation between the two methodologies, the PFC method provides more diverse information and is practiced worldwide.

As a second step, the antibody response to thymus- and macrophage-independent antigen can also be measured using similar techniques. After immunization with LPS (*Escherichia coli* lipopolysaccharide) or SSS-III (type III pneumococcal polysaccharide), the specific antibodies induced can be detected by incubating splenocytes (PFC technique) or serum (hemagglutination technique) with SRBC coated with antigen by direct adsorption (for LPS) or by coupling with a metallic agent (for SSS-III) as described by Baker *et al.* (1969). The use of hapten-conjugated T-independent antigen TNP-LPS and TNP-Ficoll (TNP, trinitrophenyl) can bring to light the precise target in the B population, that is, B cell subsets more immature (LPS) or more mature (Ficoll) (Koch *et al.,* 1982). These tests are needed only in the event of alteration of the first-step response.

A number of *in vitro* tests are also available. One of these is the immunization of dissociated spleen cells as described by Mishell and Dutton (1967). It can give a step-by-step approach for evaluating the immunotoxic effect, but it is delicate and may require addition of a metabolic activation system (a metabolite may actually be responsible for the immune defect); thus it cannot be considered as a first-approach model. Other *in vitro* tests assess the impact of a substance on the B lymphocytes: (1) lymphocyte blastogenesis induced by LPS in the mouse or by pokeweed mitogen in the rat or monkey, (2) B cell count using FITC-coated monoclonal antibodies, and (3) quantitation of the B cell progenitors (Murray *et al.,* 1983). The former is widely used but the results do not always correlate well with specific humoral responses. The latter two are both elegant but relatively expensive and for this reason can only be considered as complementary.

In summary, a good first approach is the determination of the direct PFC or evaluation of hemolysins because (1) the primary IgM response is generally more sensitive than the secondary IgG response, (2) most of the naturally occurring antigens are T dependent, and (3) these *ex vivo* tests are easy to do, rapid, inexpensive, and sensitive. They can even be too sensitive, as certain compounds devoid of any reported immune side effects in humans (such as minor tranquilizers) have been positive; inhibition in the PFC response by around 50% could be considered indicative of potential immunosuppressive activity of the drug.

E. Cell-Mediated Immunity

During the course of a cellular immune response, there is essentially a cooperation between mononuclear phagocytes (antigen-presenting cells or effectors of specific responses) and T lymphocytes. After a first antigenic stimulation, sensitized T cells respond specifically to a second contact with the antigen by releasing lymphokines. These soluble substances, such as the macrophage-inhibiting factor and interferon, are responsible for the activation of nonsensitized cells. For example, this explains the attraction of nonsensitized cells to the inflammatory site such as in tuberculin-type delayed-hypersensitivity reaction. Antigens can be proteins such as SRBC or hemocyanin, low-molecular-weight chemicals [oxazolone, dinitrochlorobenzene (DNCB)] which bind to the host proteins, and alloantigens in the case of alloreactions; in mice, macrophages present the Ia (equivalent to HLA-DR in humans) as alloantigen to the T cells which multiply, differentiate, and finally become cytotoxic T lymphocytes specifically aimed against the surface markers H-2K and H-2D (equivalent to HLA-A,B,C in humans) of the grafted cells.

For *in vivo* evaluation of delayed-type hypersensitivity (DTH), we use the footpad assay. Mice are sensitized with protein antigen injected intravenously at a very small dose (10^6 SRBC per mouse). Four days later the mice are challenged: the right foot receives the red cells whereas the left foot acts as control receiving the vehicle alone. Twenty-four hours after this second contact, the specific response is evaluated by comparing the weights of the feet sectioned at the tibiotarsal joint. Any weight difference is therefore directly due to the second presentation of the antigen. This entirely *in vivo* assay is simple, rapid, and safe. It does not use Freund's complete adjuvant (as for hemocyanin) or other sensitizing agents in humans (such as oxazolone of DNCB), nor does it need sophisticated equipment or reagents (such as the techniques that use the radiolabeling of monocyte precursors). Other data or parameters of the immune system can also be collected in parallel: white cell count, thymus and spleen weights, and histopathological findings. In addition, it is a tuberculin-type delayed hypersensitivity (Mitsuoka *et al.*, 1978; Milon *et al.*, 1983). Another approach using contact hypersensitivity to oxazolone is also very common but, for previously mentioned safety reasons, is less used in our laboratory.

Allografts are other *in vivo* models for evaluating cell-mediated immunity, grafting of either skin according to the technique of Billinghan and Medawar (1951), or allogenic tumor cells that carry the histocompatibility markers of the original mouse strain. These methods need inbred animals and consequently are most costly. Skin grafting from the C3H/He (H-2k) mouse onto the C57Bl/6 (H-2b) mouse is a very illustrative and elegant method in which the transplant is typically rejected in 10 days. However, grafting, monitoring of the animals, and daily examination of the graft starting from the seventh day are very time-consuming, and parenteral treatment of mice for the 7 days during which they still have their dressing is difficult. For these reasons, we prefer to use tumor allograft rejection, such as intraperitoneal grafting of the L1210 leukemia of DBA/2 origin (H-2d) into C3H/He mice, or subcutaneous grafting of the Sa1 sarcoma of A/J mice (H-2a) into CBA/Ca (H-2k) mice. The tumor is rejected by the immune system of the normal allogenic recipient, whereas in an immunocompromised host it grows and kills the mouse as easily as it would in a syngeneic recipient: the tumor is only used as a tool to demonstrate immunosuppression. Using the Sa1 sarcoma, rejection kinetics can be evaluated by measuring the tumor diameter every 5 days. These tumor allografts are quickly done, permit the continuation of treatment of the recipients, and are more sensitive than skin graft rejection, but they are less specific; for example, peritoneal macrophages, in the case of intraperitoneal grafting of L1210, play a role in tumor rejection of the leukemia.

One other possible *in vivo* assay is the graft versus host (GvH) reaction, where hybrid animals are injected with lymphoid cells from one parent (e.g., CBA × C57Bl/6 hybrids receiving C57Bl/6 splenocytes). In this way the grafted parental cells recognize histocompatibility markers of the other parent on the hybrid cells and thus proliferate and attack the host cells. If the cells are injected into a foot, they migrate to, and proliferate in, the popliteal lymph node (local GvH). If the cells are grafted intravenously or intraperitoneally, they induce systemic GvH, which can kill the host.

Some *in vitro* assays are also used in an attempt to evaluate a compound's impact on effector cells of the cell-mediated immunity; the effector T cells of these reactions in mice are of Ly-1 phenotype (helpers and effectors of DTH and allograft reactions) (Loveland and McKenzie, 1982) and of Ly-2,3 phenotype (cytotoxic T lymphocytes, CTL). T cell lymphocyte blastogenesis induced by T mitogens phytohemagglutinin (PHA) or concanavalin A (Con A) gives some information, which should be interpreted with caution because of the artificial conditions (compound stability in culture medium, time of exposure during blastogenesis process, etc.) and questionable correlation between response to a mitogen and cell function. Mixed-lymphocyte reaction (MLR) gives more realistic results because it mimics the reaction that takes place during allograft rejection: recognition of the foreign Ia, proliferation of helper and effector T cells (Ly-1 phenotype) in reaction to it, and then differentiation into CTL (Ly-2,3 phenotype). In these two assays cell proliferation is evaluated by tritiated-thymidine incorporation into the DNA. CTL function is quantitated by measuring CTL-mediated ^{51}Cr release from radiolabeled allogeneic target cells (tumor cells with the same H-2 markers as cells used to generate the response). The advantage of these assays is that they can be performed *ex vivo*. For example, we are trying to evaluate the lymphocyte blastogenesis response and perform some MLR in baboons during routine toxicity studies; however, these techniques have the same drawbacks as those noted above (see Section III,B, protocol conditions). They require radiolabeled compounds, sophisticated equipment, and, in the case of MLR, specific inactivation of the stimulatory cells by either X rays or mitomycin C (potential carcinogen in humans).

In conclusion, the "first-step" assay that we use for cell-mediated immunity evaluation is the footpad assay in mice. It is inexpensive, easy, and rapid to perform, and is validated using positive controls such as cyclophosphamide, corticoids (Descotes *et al.*, 1982), or enhancing agents (Bartocci *et al.*, 1982). In the event of response modifications, the precise target cells are identified in a second step by evaluating allograft rejection, lymphocyte blastogenesis induced by T mitogens and alloantigens (*ex vivo* and *in vitro* tests). These "second-step" assays are performed in conjunction with others that attempt to clarify modifications noted during other "first-step" assays such as direct PFC, resistance to *Listeria* challenge, or syngeneic tumor rejection.

F. Hypersensitivity Reactions

Specific humoral or cellular immune response in humans and animals is sometimes generated by and directed against the compound per se, but these responses induce pathological consequences in only a few cases. For example, most patients receiving penicillin produce antibodies against benzylpenicilloyl but only a few have allergic reactions (Garratty and Petz, 1975). Gell and Coombs have classified these side effects: type I (anaphylaxis), type II (antibody-mediated cytotoxicity), type III (immune complex-related disease), and type IV (delayed-type hypersensitivity). No simple animal model for predicting type II and III reactions is available. Conversely, there are specific models for the detection of type I and IV side effects, and even some widely accepted guidelines are available.

Anaphylaxis, type I reaction, is induced by various compounds such as (1) proteinaceous materials (e.g., heterologous therapeutic serum, enzymes), (2) pharmaceutical chemicals (e.g., penicillin), and (3) chemicals found in the occupational or ambient environment. The chemicals bind covalently to cellular constituents of the host and become antigenic. In the case of occupational or environmental exposure, the antigens are introduced most frequently by the respiratory route and induce allergic asthma. Type I reactions are mediated by antibodies of a particular class, the reagins (IgE). After a latency period, a subsequent contact with the product induces a very rapid response ("immediate" allergy) by the release of mediators from mast cells and basophils (such as histamine, slow-reactive substance of anaphylaxis (SRS-A), 5-hydroxytryptamine, and some prostaglandins). In the particular case of biotechnology-derived products, immunogenic trace impurities in the final product could elicit immune adverse reactions during repeated treatment of humans (insulin and growth hormone) or farm animals (bovine growth hormone and growth hormone-releasing factor analogs to improve milk or meat production). Thus, the allergenic potential of contaminants from the producing organisms (such as *Escherichia coli* proteins) and of other impurities should be assessed. The animal model used for the evaluation of potential anaphylaxis is described in detail for protein hydrolysates in European and U.S. pharmacopeiae (see reference); therefore, a full description is not given here. This test is very sensitive for proteins administered by the parenteral route, but yields little information for low-molecular-weight chemicals. In order to detect potential allergic asthma induced by occupational chemicals, inhalation of the agent itself is needed for the correct sensitization of guinea pigs (Karol, 1983; Karol *et al.*, 1985).

The guinea pig, because of its particular sensitivity, is also used for assessing a chemical's potential to induce type IV reactions, and such assessment is required by some regulatory agencies for topically applied substances, including cosmetics. Contact dermatitis is the most frequent manifestation of type IV reactions. The chemical acts as a hapten; first it binds to a skin protein or Langerhans cell membrane, then it is recognized as an immunogen, and a specific cellular immune response is triggered. After subsequent exposure, typical contact dermatitis reaction appears. This is delayed-type reaction, and for this reason, some investigators have proposed the use of Freund's complete adjuvant during the sensitization period to maximize the response, but others prefer to use repeated cutaneous applications of the compound alone because this better stimulates human exposure. These methods can be classified as (1) "maximized" methods using Freund's complete adjuvant (Magnusson and Kligman, 1969; Maurer, *et al.*, 1980) and (2) "nonmaximized" methods in which sensitization is induced by intradermal injection of the compound without adjuvant (Draize *et al.*, 1944; Landsteiner and Jacobs, 1935). The Magnusson and Kligman method is the most sensitive, whereas nonmaximized methods can only detect strong and moderate sensitizing compounds. The use of reagents such as sodium lauryl sulfate solution (Magnusson and Kligman's method) guarantees chemical penetration through the horny-layer barrier and initiates a subclinical inflammation which potentiates the allergic tissue response. A more recent method developed by Klecak *et al.* (1977) or "open epicutaneous test," which does not fit into the above classification scheme in that neither Freund's adjuvant nor intradermal injection is employed, appears to be promising; it is more sensitive than Draize's method but less than that of Magnusson and Kligman.

Particular attention should be paid to photounstable compounds, which may act as "photoantigens." On exposure to UV rays between 320 and 400 nm, they become reactive and bind to skin proteins, eliciting hypersensitivity reactions. A subsequent exposure to the product in the presence of UV rays will provoke lesions characteristic of contact dermatitis. The most well-known contact photoantigens are tribromo- and tetrachloro-salicylanilides which were used as germicides in soap and were responsible for severe contact dermatitis in humans; they are excellent positive controls in guinea pigs (Harber *et al.*, 1967). This concept of photoallergy can be extended to other exposure routes as shown for some sulfonamides (Burckhardt, 1948), chlorpromazine, or amiodarone hydrochloride. With the latter compound, patient photosensitivity persists after withdrawal because of lipid storage of the compound (Unkovic *et al.*, 1984).

In summary, certain compounds, because of chemical structure and/or administration route, could be suspected of inducing allergic responses, and testing is required by regulatory agencies. The tests are well standardized and relatively predictive, and they should be part of a routine toxicity testing program.

G. Realistic Criteria for Immunotoxicity Assessment

The investigation of possible immunotoxicological effects of a new compound is begun by considering which tests to choose and when to perform them. The answers lie in the (1) chemical structure and physicochemical properties, (2) type of therapeutic agent, (3) alarm signals observed during toxicity testing, and, of course, (4) governmental guidelines if available. Examples given below illustrate this approach.

Physicochemical characteristics of a compound can point to possible immune side effects. Photoallergenic substances are photounstable compounds particularly sensitive to the UV spectrum between 320 and 400 nm. Any compound which markedly absorbs in this range is a possible photoallergen, and, thus, its photoallergenic potential should be evaluated early in its development, even if not intended for topical administration.

Therapeutic agents intended to act on the immune system, such as immunomodulating agents or immunotoxins (complexes made up of a monoclonal antibody and a cytotoxic agent, such as ricin or gelonin), have already had their impact on this system assessed during pharmacology studies. Therefore, the immunotoxicologist is concerned rather with indirect side effects. For example, with immunotoxins, the link between antibody and toxin can be broken either during storage or *in vivo,* and the toxin released; thus it is important to evaluate the effect of the toxin per se because these toxins have immunosuppressive capacities (Spreafico *et al.*, 1983; Descotes *et al.*, 1985). Toxicological evaluation of the anti-T-lymphocyte immunotoxin T101 (ricin A-chain plus monoclonal antibody T101) parenterally administered to rats or macaque monkeys for 5 days was accompanied by polysynovitis and biological inflammatory changes related more to repeated injection of high-molecular-weight foreign protein complex than to the pharmacological activity of the complex.

Another example of the importance of considering the therapeutic class of agents in selecting tests is given by anticancer compounds that are cytotoxic and often myelotoxic. Myelotoxic effects of such compounds should be evaluated at the first stages of the routine toxicity testing. The Till and McCulloch (1961) approach could be used initially. It differentiates between a simple cytotoxicity as with cyclophosphamide, and cytotoxicity affecting also pluripotent stem cell capacity to generate colonies (colony-forming units, CFU) as with busulfan. Further evaluation of different cell line precursors (CFU-E for erythrocytes, CFU-GM for mononuclear phagocytes and granulocytes, CFU-M for megakaryocytes and platelets) requires special experimental conditions. Performed *ex vivo* and/or *in vitro,* these tests are more delicate and in practice are undertaken later or only in the case of unexpected cytopenia observed during toxicity studies.

When numerous scientific papers report immune side effects of certain families of agents, toxicity testing of related compounds should include immunotoxicological tests. For example, the immune system, like the gastrointestinal tract or the kidney, could be one of the targets of antiinflammatory or antiarthritic agents. In this case, the tests should be performed before multiple-dose clinical trials and could consist of (1) resistance to an experimental infection, (2) rejection of a syngeneic tumor, (3) antibody response to a T-dependent antigen, and (4) DTH reaction. Each assay should include two types of positive controls: a compound of the same therapeutic class at dose levels pharmacologically comparable and a well-known immunomodulating agent to validate the experiment.

As these examples show, a rigid approach cannot be used to evaluate immunotoxic potential. The approach must be elaborated on a case-by-case basis taking into account the compound characteristics, stage of development, and data from other studies (pharmacokinetics and routine toxicity). In the particular case of the "human" products obtained by recombinant DNA technology, classical toxicity testing in animals may sometimes bring to light adverse effects mediated by the host cell contaminants or even by the vehicle (Matory *et al.,* 1985). Conversely, this approach often fails to detect intrinsic toxicity of the compound (Schellekens *et al.,* 1984) and furthermore could be accompanied by an associated species-specific immune response against the compound per se (including neutralizing antibodies and/or immune-related pathologies). Thus the laboratory should be prepared to look at not only anticontaminants but also antiproduct antibodies.

H. Examples of Immune Side Effects Observed during Toxicity Studies

Below are two examples of side effects observed during toxicity studies and mediated by or directed toward the immune system.

1. Circulating Immune Complex-Related Disease

A few compounds (antibiotics) have been reported to produce glomerular nephritis in humans. During routine toxicity testing of a new β-lactam antibiotic in baboons (i.v. route, 150–600 mg/kg daily), typical signs of circulating immune complex (CIC)-related pathology were observed the fourth week of treatment in some animals without a dose-related pattern.

Characteristic clinical signs were palpebral, submandibular, and ventral subcutaneous edema, palpebral purpura, hypoalbuminemia followed by hypoproteinemia, increased BUN and creatinine levels, and proteinuria. Autopsy revealed ascites and large pale kidneys with red spots on the cortex. Histopathological examination confirmed glomerular injury: focal and segmentary glomerular nephritis with vacuolization of epithelial cells and formation of crescents, and subacute inflammation taking the form of periarteriolar cuffings Complementary examinations confirmed these observations: irregular deposits on the glomerular basement membrane suggesting immune complexes were seen by electron microscopy, and glomerular, granular discontinuous fluorescence was observed by direct immunofluorescence technique using anti-IgG antiserum. Also, circulating immune complexes were determined in serum samples (collected during the study and stored in deep-freeze) by ELISA according to Manca *et al.* (1980). In this technique, *E. coli* β-galactosidase anti–β-galactosidase probe immune complex competes with baboon serum CIC for bovine conglutinin adsorbed on polystyrene beads through C3bi complement fraction, and level of enzyme activity on the solid phase is measured by hydrolysis of the enzyme substrate. Figure 1 shows an example of the CIC level over time in a treated baboon: demonstrating increase in the CIC levels prior to any biochemical changes and subsequent decrease prior to death.

2. *Dyslipidic Thesaurismosis*

Numerous amphiphilic cationic compounds cause lipid lysosomal storage (or dyslipidic thesaurismosis) in animal and sometimes in human tissues; one of these is amiodarone hydrochloride, a unique antiarrhythmic agent. Toxicity studies conducted with amiodarone showed that sublethal doses (up to 100–150 mg/kg/day), administered by gavage for 4 weeks, induced lipid storage in a variety of rat tissues, which was strain dependent (Fischer-sensitive and Wistar-resistant). Under similar treatment, beagle dogs developed a similar reaction, whereas baboons did not. In sensitive animals, Peyer's patches and mesenteric lymph nodes were the first invaded, then the remaining lymph nodes and other organs, particularly the lung. Light-microscopic examination revealed, in apparently lymphocyte-depleted lymph nodes, distended foamy macrophages with vacuolated cytoplasm and prepyknotic nuclei. On electron microscopy, these foam cells (including

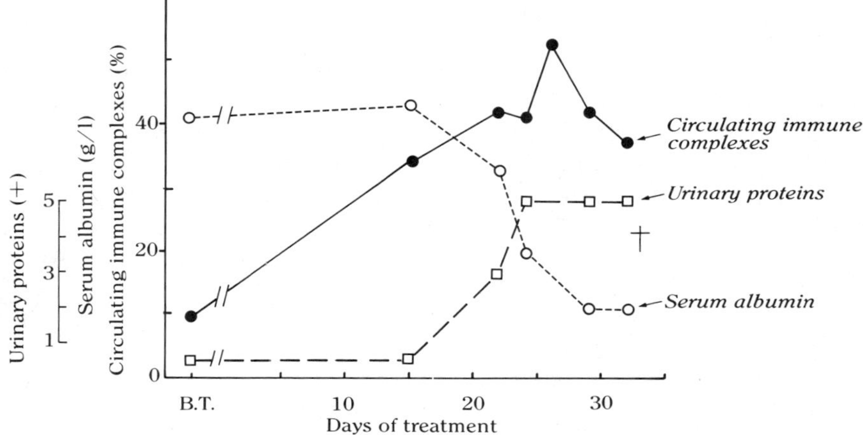

FIG. 1. Serum albumin, circulating immune complex, and urinary protein levels in a baboon receiving daily i.v. administration of a new β-lactam antibiotic. Urinary protein levels measured using AMES Multistix. B.T., Before treatment; cross at day 32 indicates death of animal.

alveolar macrophages harvested by bronchoalveolar lavage) were filled with numerous concentrically lamellated complexes. In order to correlate these morphological changes with possible functional alterations, immunotoxicity studies were performed; inbred (C57Bl/6 and C3H/He) or outbred (Swiss) mice were treated by gavage for 1 month at dose levels up to 200 mg/kg/day, and immune reactions requiring macrophage activities were then evaluated. Neither resistance to *Listeria* challenge, nor specific humoral (PFC assay) or cellular (footpad assay) immune responses were altered. These findings are in accordance with those described in humans on long-term treatment: lipid storage in the corneal epithelium (D'Amico *et al.*, 1981) and diffuse interstitial pneumopathy (Sobol and Rakita, 1982) without any functional injury of the immune system have been reported.

IV. Conclusion

The immune system is essential to the survival of the higher organisms, and, thus, safety evaluation of xenobiotics must take into account effects on this system, from the routine toxicity testing to specific immunological tests. Awareness of the importance of immunotoxicity testing has been growing only in recent years, and few regulatory guidelines are currently available, but more will undoubtedly be forthcoming in the near future.

Of primary concern is the choice of tests and timing. Validated immunopharmacological tests are available, of which a few are applied to evaluate the immunotoxicological potential of xenobiotics. First-step assays are reliable indicators of general events in humans or animals; however, further testing is required to identify precise target cells in the immune system.

Based on our experience in the field of pharmaceutical industry, we recommend, for therapeutic classes reported to have no impact on the immune system, the analysis of data from classical toxicity studies. Only if data show or suggest an effect, are specific tests conducted to confirm the findings and, in the case of effect, to identify the nature of the immune system damage. Where the compound studied belongs to a class with known effects on the immune system, the risk:benefit ratio must be evaluated by comparison with a well-studied member of that class. Finally, for a new compound about which little is known, as a precaution, immunotoxicity assays should first be performed before repeated administrations for more than 1 week in humans.

Acknowledgments

We thank L. Olsen, H. Delon, and M. Jones for their patience and help in preparing the manuscript.

References

Baker, P. J., Stashak, P. W., and Prescott, B. (1969). *Appl. Microbiol.* **17,** 422–426.

Bartocci, A., Read, E. L., Welker, R. D., Schlick, E., Papademetriou, V., and Chirigos, M. A. (1982). *Cancer Res.* **43,** 3514–3518.

Billinghan, R. E., and Medawar, P. B. (1951). *J. Exp. Biol.* **28,** 385–389.

Boorman, G. A., Luster, M. I., Dean, J. H., and Wilson, R. E. (1980). *J. Reticuloendothel. Soc.* **28,** 547–559.

Boorman, G. A., Luster, M. I., Dean, J. H., Campbell, M. L., Lauer, L. D., Talley, F. A., Wilson, R. E., and Collins, M. J. (1982). *Am. J. Pathol.* **106,** 110–117.

Burckhardt, W. (1948). *Dermatologica* **96,** 280–285.

Burnet, F. M. (1970). *Prog. Exp. Tumor Res.* **13,** 1–27.

Cunningham, A. J., and Szenberg, A. (1968). *Immunology* **14,** 599–601.

D'Amico, D. J., Kenyon, K. R., and Ruskin, J. N. (1981). *Arch. Ophtalmol.* **99,** 257–261.

Dean, J. H., Padarathsingh, M. L., and Jerrels, T. R. (1979a). *Drug Chem. Toxicol.* **2,** 5–17.

Dean, J. H., Padarathsingh, M. L., Jerrells, T. R., Keys, L., and Northing, J. W. (1979b). *Drug Chem. Toxicol.* **2,** 133–153.

Dean, J. H., Luster, M. I., Boorman, G. A., Luebke, R. W., and Lauer, L. D. (1980). *J. Reticuloendothel. Soc.* **28,** 571–583.

Dean, J. H., Luster, M. I., Murray, M. J., and Lauer, L. D. (1983). *In* "Immunotoxicology" (G. Gibson, R. Hubbard, and R. Parke, eds.), pp. 205–218. Academic Press, London.
Descotes, G., Mazué, G., and Richez, P. (1982). *Toxicol. Lett.* **13,** 129–138.
Descotes, G., Romano, M., Stirpe, F., and Spreafico, F. (1985). *Int. J. Immunopharmacol.* **7,** 455–463.
Draize, J. H., Woodhard, G., and Calvery, H. O. (1944). *J. Pharmacol. Exp. Ther.* **82,** 377–390.
Fish, L. A., Baxter, C. S., and Bash, J. A. (1981). *Toxicology* **19,** 127–138.
Garratty, G., and Petz, L. D. (1975). *Am. J. Med.* **58,** 398–407.
Gresser, I., Tovey, M. G., Maury, C., and Bandu, M. T. (1976). *J. Exp. Med.* **144,** 1316–1323.
Hanna, N., and Burton, R. C. (1981). *J. Immunol.* **127,** 1754–1758.
Harber, L. C., Targovnik, S. E., and Baer, R. L. (1967). *Arch. Dermatol.* **96,** 646–656.
Herbermann, R. B., ed. (1982). "NK Cells and Other Effector Cells." Academic Press, New York.
Hurtrel, B., Lagrange, P. H., and Michel, J.-C. (1980). *Ann. Immunol. (Inst. Pasteur)* **131C,** 105–118.
Jerne, N. K., and Nordin, A. A. (1963). *Science* **140,** 405.
Karol, M. H. (1983). *Toxicol. Appl. Pharmacol.* **68,** 229–241.
Karol, M. H., Stadler, J., and Magreni, C. (1985). *Fundam. Appl. Toxicol.* **5,** 459–472.
Keller, R. (1979). *Nature (London)* **282,** 729–731.
Kern, E. R. (1982). *Environ. Health Perspect.* **43,** 71–79.
Klecak, G., Geleick, H., and Frey, J. R. (1977). *J. Soc. Cosmet. Chem.* **28,** 53–64.
Koch, G., Lok, B. D., Van Oudenaren, A., and Benner, R. (1982). *J. Immunol.* **128,** 1497–1501.
Landsteiner, K., and Jacobs, J. (1935). *J. Exp. Med.* **61,** 643–655.
Larsch, J. E., Race, G. J., Martin, J. H., and Weatherly, N. F. (1974). *J. Parasitol.* **60,** 99–109.
Loveland, B. E., and McKenzie, I. F. C. (1982). *Transplantation* **33,** 217–221.
Luster, M. I., and Faith, R. E. (1979). *Ann. N.Y. Acad. Sci.* **320,** 572–578.
Magnusson, B., and Kligman, A. M. (1969). *J. Invest. Dermatol.* **52,** 268–276.
Manca, F., Migliorini, P., Bombardieri, S., and Celada, F. (1980). *Clin. Immunol. Immunopathol.* **16,** 131–141.
Mantovani, A., Luini, W., Peri, G., Vecci, A., and Spreafico, F. (1978). *J. Natl. Cancer Inst.* **61,** 1255–1261.
Matory, Y. L., Chang, A. E., Lipford, E. H., Braziel, R., Hyatt, C. L., McDonald, H. D., and Rosenberg, S. A. (1986). *J. Biol. Response Mod.* **4,** 377–390.
Maurer, T., Weirich, E. G., and Hess, R. (1980). *Toxicology* **15,** 163–171.
Milon, G., Marchal, G., Seman, M., Truffa-Bachi, P., and Zilberfarb, V. (1983). *J. Immunol.* **130,** 1103–1107.
Mishell, R. I., and Dutton, R. W. (1967). *J. Exp. Med.* **126,** 423–442.
Mitsuoka, A., Teramatsu, T., Baba, M., Morikawa, S., and Yasuhira, K. (1978). *Immunology* **34,** 363–370.
Morahan, P. S., Klykken, P. C., Smith, S. H., Harris, L. S., and Munson, A. (1979). *Infect. Immun.* **23,** 670–674.
Murray, M. J., Wilson, F. D., Fisher, G. L., and Erickson, K. L. (1983). *Clin. Exp. Immunol.* **53,** 744–749.
Murray, M. J., Lauer, L. D., Luster, M. I., Luebke, R. W., Adams, D. O., and Dean, J. H. (1985). *Int. J. Immunopharmacol.* **7,** 491–500.
Penn, I. (1978). *Adv. Surg.* **12,** 155–191.

Riccardi, C., Puccetti, P., Santoni, A., and Herberman, R. B. (1979). *J. Natl. Cancer Inst.* **63,** 1041–1045.
Schellekens, H., De Reus, A., and von den Meide, P. H. (1984). *J. Med. Primatol.* **13,** 235–245.
Sobol, S. ., and Rakita, L. (1982). *Circulation* **65,** 819–824.
Spreafico, F., Malfiore, C., Moras, M. L., Marmonti, L., Filippeschi, S., Barbieri, L., Perocco, P., and Stirpe, F. (1983). *Int. J. Immunopharmacol.* **5,** 335–343.
Till, J. E., and McCulloch, E. A. (1961). *Radiat. Res.* **14,** 213–222.
Tripathy, S. P., and Mackaness, G. B. (1969). *J. Exp. Med.* **130,** 1–16.
Unkovic, J., Combes, M., Mazué, G., and Roncucci, R. (1984). *Poster Annu. Meet. Am. Soc. Dermatol., 43rd, Washington, D.C. Dec. 1–6.*
U.S. Pharmacopeia (1985). 21st Ed., pp. 911–912.
Vecchi, A., Sironi, M., Canegrati, M. A., Recchia, M., and Garattini, S. (1983). *Toxicol. Appl. Pharmacol.* **68,** 434–441.
Vos, J. G. (1977). *CRC Crit. Rev. Toxicol.* **5,** 67–101.
Winkelstein, J. A., and Swift, A. J. (1975). *Infect. Immun.* **12,** 1222–1223.

The Endocrine System as the Target in Experimental Toxicology

F. X. R. VAN LEEUWEN,* M. A. M. FRANKEN,†
AND J. G. LOEBER‡

*Laboratories for *Toxicology, †Pathology, and ‡Clinical Chemistry,
The National Institute of Public Health and Environmental Hygiene,
3720 BA Bilthoven, The Netherlands*

I. Introduction

Besides the nervous system and the immune system, the endocrine system is an important integrating system in the mammalian body. Its principal action is to control the metabolic functions (Guyton, 1976). The endocrine organs maintain homeostasis, regulate growth, maturation, and reproductive processes, and have the capacity to react to external stimuli. All these processes act via a complex network of hormonal interactions, responses, and feedback mechanisms. As a result of the fine-regulated hormonal interactions, the endocrine system may be particularly vulnerable to the effects of toxic compounds, and, subsequently, dysfunction of the endocrine system may lead to a broad variety of effects as can be found in toxicological studies. A common observation such as delayed growth or metabolic dysfunction may be the result of decreased thyroid function, due to a direct interaction of toxic agents with the thyroid gland or mediated via a decreased thyrotropin (TSH) release by the pituitary gland. Alterations of carbohydrate metabolism in the liver may also be due to pancreatic dysfunction. Toxic compounds sometimes disturb kidney function directly by interference with glomerular or tubular filtration processes, but similar effects can also be due to variations in hormonal regulation, mediated, for instance, by the adrenal glands. With decreased fertility or reproductive performance, it is obvious that the gonads are the target organs. In these cases changes in biosynthesis, release, or response of sex steroids might be the underlying mechanism.

Extension of the knowledge of endocrine toxicology is also important with respect to the understanding of sex-linked differences in the onset and expression of toxicological phenomena, as observed with many compounds. In addition, it should be mentioned that an enhanced hormonal stimulation frequently leads to nonneoplastic growth in endocrine organs like the pituitary and thyroid glands, pancreas, and gonads, sometimes resulting in tumor formation, and that in some cases hormones promote the proliferation of tumor cells in target organs (IARC, 1979). Via this endocrine mechanism, exogenous as well as endogenous compounds can act as tumor promoters, and it is imperative for toxicologists to distinguish this latter mechanism of action from a direct genotoxic action. Also in this particular field, endocrine toxicology can provide additional information which is extremely relevant.

Very often endocrine toxicology is an essential extension of routine toxicity testing. Incorporation of endocrine parameters in toxicological studies is important not only to reveal the mechanism of action of exogenous compounds in hormonal target cells, but also to enable investigators to establish a sensitive and relevant "no-effect level," which is necessary for a reliable risk evaluation of endocrine toxins.

In relation to the relevance of endocrine toxicology, as mentioned above, it is amazing that in routine toxicity testing hardly any attention is paid to the endocrine system. In the past, lack of specific and sensitive methods and test materials might have been the main reason why toxicologists more or less restricted their investigations to morphological changes in endocrine organs or the detection of overall alterations like weight changes or disturbances of the reproductive performance. However, the development of species-specific antibodies has greatly expanded the potential of unraveling the interactions of chemical compounds with the endocrine system. At present it is possible to determine a variety of hormones in tissue fluids of various species by radioimmunoassay (RIA) or enzyme-linked immunosorbent assay (ELISA). Hormone-producing cells in various endocrine organs can be easily and specifically detected in tissue sections by immunocytochemistry, and, furthermore, disturbance of the function of endocrine organs can be determined with specific function tests. These methods provide a suitable panel of tools to tackle the problems of endocrine toxicology in routine toxicity testing, so that a no-effect level based upon endocrine alterations can be derived.

In this chapter we stress the importance of endocrine toxicology, discuss some practical problems, describe methods of investigation, and show some examples of endocrine toxicological experiments.

II. No-Hormonal-Effect Level

The concept of the "no-hormonal-effect level (NHEL)" was introduced recently during the international discussions dealing with the safety evaluation of anabolic agents. In principle the term "no-hormonal-effect level" was used to define the no-effect level of exogenous (as well as endogenous) anabolic agents, in other words "a no-effect level of a compound with hormonal activity." In fact, this means a compound that interferes with the endocrine system on a level of hormone–receptor interactions and response.

For anabolic agents, estrogens as well as androgens, special toxicological test systems have been developed to establish a no-effect level. The results obtained with some anabolic agents in these test systems, are described in detail by Foxcroft and Hess (1986). It appeared from the results of *in vivo* tests with intact and ovariectomized monkeys treated with estrogens, and intact and castrated monkeys and pigs treated with androgens, that a unique and sensitive set of tests was available for the establishment of a NHEL (Parekh and Coulston, 1983; Foxcroft, 1983; Hess, 1983). However, these tests had been developed in particular for a small group of hormonal active compounds, and the question arises whether the concept of the NHEL can find a broader and more general application. In general, a NHEL can be defined as a "no-effect level of any compound altering endocrine function." With this definition it does not matter whether this occurs via a direct hormonal interaction, such as the interference with receptor interactions as is the case for anabolic agents, or whether the compound exerts its effect on the endocrine system via an indirect mechanism like (1) alteration in biosynthesis of hormones, (2) interference with uptake of hormones or their precursors, (3) interference with hormone release, (4) alteration in metabolic breakdown of hormones, or (5) interaction with the second-messenger (cAMP) system. Whenever an exogenous compound exerts its toxic effect via one of the above-mentioned mechanisms, it also might lead to a disturbance of the function of the endocrine system, sometimes leading to a prominent toxic effect.

In order to study these effects, endocrine parameters should be incorporated in toxicity testing. A logical and reliable strategy, particularly in short-term (e.g., subacute and subchronic) but also in long-term *in vivo* studies, is a combined morphological and biochemical approach (Table I). It starts with the determination of the weight of endocrine organs and histological appearance of these organs, more or less as screening parameters. If there are indications of disturbances in the endocrine system, the next step is the determination of circulating

TABLE I

METHODS TO DETECT ENDOCRINE ALTERATIONS IN TOXICITY TESTING

Type of method	Examples
Screening	Endocrine organ weights Histology (light microscopy)
Specific	Immunoassays (RIA) Enzyme- and immunocytochemistry (light and electron microscopy) Function studies (uptake, release and inhibitory tests) Ectomy (adrenalectomy, gonadectomy–feedback interactions) *In vitro* methods (cell or tissue culture, receptor interactions)

hormones, possibly in combination with specific morphological or immunocytochemical methods. As the next step, specific function tests like release tests and biochemical methods establishing dysfunction of particular endocrine organs can be carried out. By ectomy, the involvement of particular endocrine organs can be examined. Finally, *in vitro* methods can be used to establish the mechanism of action. This type of strategy offers insight in the target organ(s), the level of interaction, and the mechanism by which toxic compounds interfere with endocrine function.

III. Practical Considerations

One of the first problems one encounters in endocrine toxicology is the choice of the animal species. In routine toxicity testing the rat is the species most frequently used. Over the years the rat has served also as an excellent model in studies of endocrine mechanisms. Furthermore, various rat-specific antisera of tropic hormones can be obtained from the National Institute of Arthritis, Diabetes and Digestive and Kidney Diseases (NIADDK), Bethesda, Maryland, via the Rat Pituitary Hormone Distribution Program. Details can be found in the January and July issues (1985) of the periodicals *Endocrinology,* and *Journal of Endocrinology and Metabolism*. Thus endocrine effects can be studied in conjunction with overall toxicity in the same animal species. However, it can be questioned if the rat always is the most appropriate species for endocrine toxicity testing.

Nonhuman primates like rhesus or cynomolgus monkeys have also been advocated by the Food and Drug Administration as appropriate animals to study estrogenic compounds. This is primarily based on the resemblance in estrous cycle between these animals and human beings, which is regarded as an advantage in extrapolating animal data for human risk assessment.

For investigations of toxic effects other than on the gonads, male animals may be more appropriate than females, due to the absence of interference of the estrous cycle with basal metabolic and endocrine processes. There is evidence that the developing endocrine system in immature animals is much more susceptible to toxic compounds than the mature one. This holds for direct effects on the gonads as well as for thyroid dysfunction accompanied by functional alterations in the pituitary–gonadal axis, for example. This favors the use of weanling or immature animals in short-term endocrine toxicity testing. However, one encounters difficulties in manipulating young animals, in particular with respect to cannulation of blood vessels for sampling procedures.

Results in endocrine toxicology may be confounded by variations in hormonal data due to animal stress and variations in housing conditions, diet, and sampling procedures. Therefore, in general, experimental conditions should be standardized to reduce these variations as much as possible. It has long been known that laboratory animals, in particular some rat strains, are very sensitive to external stimuli (stress factors), which affect a large number of endocrine parameters in the circulation (Barrett and Stockham, 1963). Among these parameters, those of the hypothalamic–pituitary–adrenal axis are the most prominent. Stress leads to increased concentrations of corticotropin-releasing hormone (CRH or corticoliberin), adrenocorticotropic hormone (ACTH or corticotropin), and corticosteroids, respectively. In addition, stress yields a pronounced increase of prolactin and a sharp decrease of growth hormone. For obvious reasons it is necessary to avoid stress as much as possible. The main causes of stress are handling, transport, and noise (Döhler *et al.*, 1977; Krulich *et al.*, 1974). The first cause can be reduced by daily and frequent handling of the animals during the experimental period so that they become accustomed to manipulating procedures. The last two factors can usually be kept to a minimum by moving the rats from their quarters to the laboratory well in advance of the sampling procedure. Absolute silence during sampling is essential. Hissing sounds as rustling paper and running tap water are to be especially avoided.

For the sampling itself the animals usually have to be manipulated. Quick decapitation without anesthesia is an efficient way to obtain blood and results in less stress compared to cardiac, retroorbital sinus, or abdominal aorta puncture under ether, chloroform, or Nembutal anesthesia (Döhler *et al.,* 1977). A drawback may be that the sample is contaminated with some other body fluids. Moreover, such organs as the thyroid gland and the lungs may be damaged, rendering them unsuitable for subsequent histological examination. For ethical reasons, other methods of blood sampling such as orbital puncture or cutting of the tail tip commonly are carried out under light anesthesia. However, as mentioned above, anesthetics exert considerable influences on the endocrine system and are therefore less suitable.

An elegant way to overcome these negative aspects is cannulation of a major blood vessel such as the vena jugularis or the vena iliaca. This is commonly achieved under ether or pentobarbital anesthesia at least 1 day before the sampling. Several procedures have been described (Steffens, 1969; Andrews and Ojeda, 1981; Mattheij and Van Pijkeren, 1984). Briefly, a silicon rubber cannula, which is inserted into the vein and moved up to such a position that the internal tip just reaches the right atrium, is moved subcutaneously to the back of the skull and fixed there. By connecting a syringe to this system via an external catheter, it is possible to sample blood at any desired moment. This latter is important, since for a proper evaluation of endocrine parameters establishment of baseline levels of circulating hormones in the selected species or strain is necessary. Biological parameters, and in particular hormone concentrations, are influenced by a natural periodicity. This depends on a series of factors like the changing of seasons, the sleep–wake cycle, and the diurnal or circadian rhythm (Döhler and Wuttke, 1976; Wisser and Breuer, 1981). These biological rhythms result in daily fluctuations of test results. By selecting the proper sampling time, these fluctuations can be reduced with a consequent increase in resolution of the test. So by cannulation of the animals, the problems associated with stress and circadian rhythms can be overcome. This system also offers the opportunity for intravenous administration of any compound to the animal; hence, function tests can be performed relatively simply.

Fluctuations in hormonal parameters may also occur as a result of the interaction between the endocrine and immune systems. Growth hormone (GH), a thymotropic hormone, affects the function of thymus and peripheral lymphoid organs; estrogens and androgens are involved in various immune alterations, and glucocorticoids play a role in lymphocyte function (Cupps and Fauci, 1982; Luster *et al.,* 1985; Vos, 1977). Any stimulation (e.g., by a pathogenic organism) of the host's defense system may result in endocrine alterations, this being an important reason to carry out endocrine toxicological experiments with specific pathogen-free (SPF) animals, held under a rigid sanitary regimen.

In endocrine toxicology specific requirements with respect to the composition of the animal diet are essential. Purity, type, and amount of all food commodities like nutrients and minerals must be well defined. Adequate amounts of calcium, phosphate, and magnesium are important with respect to optimal calcitonin–parathyroid hormone mechanisms, in particular in relation with sex-linked nephrocalcinosis in Wistar rats (Harwood, 1982). Potassium and sodium must be present in an adequate amount in relation to mineralocorticoid secretion and iodine in relation to thyroid function. In general it can be stated that excess of the above-mentioned compounds can mask effects of toxic compounds whereas inadequacy enhances the effects. Depending on the source of the diet, goitrogens (Liener, 1979) or estrogens (Rackis, 1974) can be present, disturbing "normal" endocrine functioning. Also, the amount and composition of proteins, carbohydrates, and lipids is of importance, since they interfere with thyroid, pancreatic, and adrenal function, respectively (Singh *et al.*, 1971; Maji *et al.*, 1980; Lawson *et al.*, 1981). Therefore information about dietary composition is a basal requirement for relevant endocrine toxicology.

IV. Applied Techniques

A. Histological Methods

First indications of chemically induced modifications of the endocrine system may be obtained from weight changes and histopathological alterations. Although the routine histological staining procedures, such as hematoxylin and eosin staining, are very useful for the identification of an endocrine toxic compound, these do not elucidate the level at which the endocrine system has been affected, including the biosynthetic pathway of hormones, the number of specific hormone-producing cells present, and the cellular hormone content. Advances in the field of enzyme histochemistry, immunocytochemistry, and electron microscopy have yielded highly sensitive and specific techniques for the localization of a variety of enzyme activities and hormones in tissue sections. Prerequisites for these methods are proper fixation and processing procedures of the tissue.

1. Enzyme Cytochemistry

With this method, sites of enzymatic activity are visualized through a colored insoluble precipitate by incubating tissue sections in a medium containing the appropriate substrate, coenzymes, and cofactors. In endocrine toxicology, enzyme histochemistry has proved to be valuable for the demonstration of the activities of important steroidogenic enzymes or enzymes indicating steroidogenic cellular sites (Shivanandappa and Krishnakumari, 1983). Unfixed cryostat sections of tissue frozen in liquid nitrogen are commonly used, although the cytological detail is less than optimal. At the electron-microscopic level, steroidogenic enzymatic activity in rat adrenals has been demonstrated with an acceptable conservation of the tissue structure (Berchtold, 1977).

2. *Immunocytochemistry*

In general, immunocytochemical methods have the great advantage that many antigens—for example, hormones—can be demonstrated through an antigen–antibody reaction using a marker conjugated with the antibody. The aim of these methods is the achievement of intense staining, minimal nonspecific background staining, and sufficient sensitivity to stain the cells with high dilutions of the antiserum. In immunofluorescence using frozen cryostat sections, markers such as isothiocyanates of fluorescein (FITC) and, to a lesser extent, of tetramethylrhodamine (TRITC) are employed, being directly visible under the fluorescence microscope. In paraffin sections of formalin-fixed tissue, enzyme markers including horseradish peroxidase, glucose oxidase, and alkaline phosphatase are widely used and visualized by addition of a substrate solution which reacts with the enzyme label to an insoluble staining product. Electron-dense markers such as ferritin and colloidal gold enable the localization of antigens at the ultrastructural level.

Of the enzyme markers mentioned, horseradish peroxidase is by far the most applied, because its conjugation with immunoglobulins is rather easy without much impairment of activity. Moreover, many chromogenic substrates for peroxidase are available (e.g., diaminobenzidine) which yield an insoluble colored product that is visible on light microscopy and, after chelation with osmium, also on electron microscopy. Various immunoperoxidase techniques are accessible, including the peroxidase-labeled antibody method (of which there are both direct and indirect versions (Nakane and Pierce, 1966), the unlabeled antibody method of peroxidase–antiperoxidase (PAP) (Sternberger, 1979), and the avidin–biotin–peroxidase complex (ABC) method (Hsu *et al.*, 1981). By addition of compounds such as imidazole, the cytochemical reaction for peroxidase can be enhanced (Straus, 1982).

The indirect peroxidase-labeled antibody method is most commonly used in our toxicity studies with rats when a compound appears to influence the endocrine system. The pituitary gland plays a central role in the endocrine system, producing several tropic hormones. With the conventional histological hematoxylin and eosin staining, in the rat anterior pituitary gland three types of cells can be discriminated, namely, acidophilic, basophilic, and chromophobic cells. The glycoproteins constitute two subunits, α and β. The α subunits correspond, while the β subunits are specific for structure and function of each hormone. By application of immunoperoxidase techniques, the different hormone-producing cells can be specifically localized. Antisera against pituitary hormones are usually species-specific. Many of the rat antisera were obtained from the NIADDK (Bethesda, Maryland). Using the indirect peroxidase-labeled antibody method of Nakane and Pierce (1966), with 3,3′-diaminobenzidine and hydrogen peroxide as substrates for peroxidase (Graham and Karnovsky, 1966), selective immunocytochemical staining could be localized in different cell types in the anterior pituitary gland of rats, fixed in formalin-sublimate and embedded in paraplast. Immunoreactive GH-producing cells were seen to be scattered throughout the anterior lobe, frequently forming small clusters or strings. The cytoplasm was strongly stained and the cells were round to oval in shape (Fig. 1). The prolactin (PRL) cells revealed with anti-PRL serum were also seen homogeneously distributed throughout the pars anterior, being cup-shaped in the females (Fig. 2a) or stellate in the males (Fig. 2b). Many stellate cells with interdigitating cytoplasmic processes were positive for ACTH and were preferentially localized in the lateral parts of the anterior pituitary (Fig. 2c). TSH-producing cells appeared to be polygonal, mainly located in the central part of the anterior lobe. They were more or less intensely stained (Fig. 2d). In the rat, immunoreactivity for luteinizing hormone (LH) and follicle-stimulating hormone (FSH) was localized predominantly in the same gonadotropic cells, showing both strong and weak reactions. The immunoreactive FSH and LH cells in the females as well as the FSH cells in the males were present throughout the anterior pituitary gland, whereas the strongly immunoreactive LH cells in the males were more concentrated in the caudolateral areas. The cells had round to polygonal shapes (Fig. 2e and f).

Apart from immunoperoxidase methods, electron-microscopic techniques make use of electron-dense markers such as ferritin and especially colloidal gold. The high molecular weight of ferritin, however, hampers its penetration into the cells, so it is mostly employed for the localization of membrane-associated antigens. The introduction of the immunogold reagent (i.e., immunoglobulin adsorbed to the surface of colloidal gold particles) has greatly facilitated the visualization of

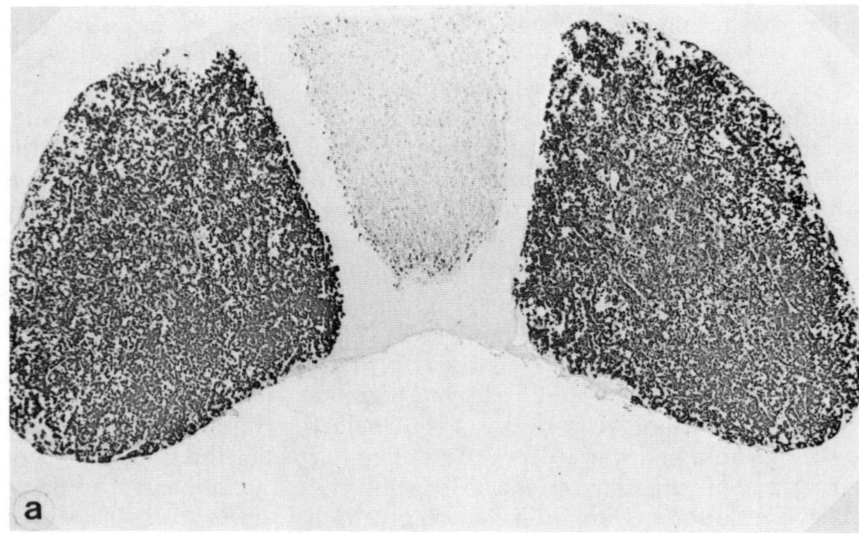

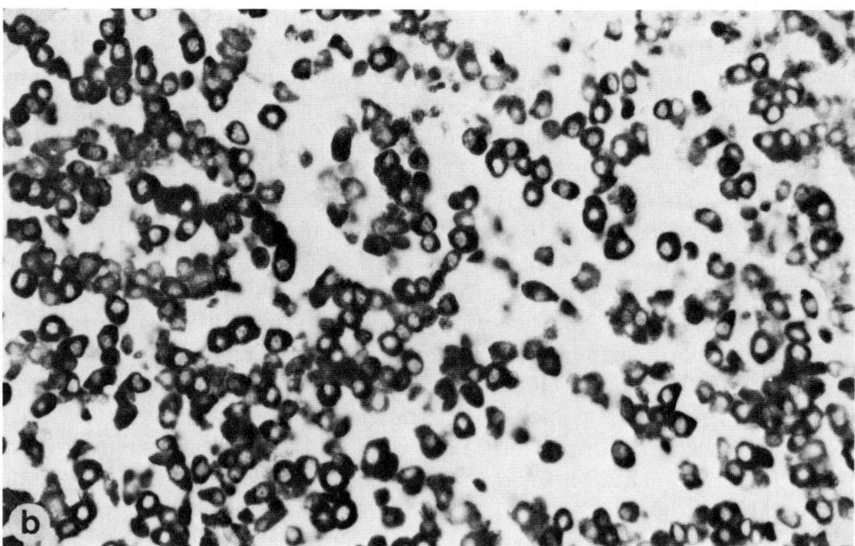

FIG. 1. Immunocytochemical staining (indirect peroxidase-labeled antibody method) for GH in the pituitary gland of an adult untreated rat. (a) Overall picture (×30) showing immunoreactive GH cells to be localized specifically in the anterior lobe (AL) compared to the intermediate lobe (IL) and the posterior lobe (PL). (b) Detail of (a) showing the immunoreactive GH cells forming small clusters or strings and round to oval in shape. ×300.

various intracellular antigenic sites on thin sections (Faulk and Taylor, 1971). Moreover, complexes of colloidal gold with staphylococcal protein A, which reacts specifically with the Fc fragment of IgG molecules, has become of special interest (Romano and Romano, 1977). Incubation of the sections with a specific antiserum is then followed by visualization of the antigen–IgG complex through the protein A–gold solution. The use of gold particles of different diameter enables double labeling at the subcellular level (Geuze *et al.*, 1981).

For light-microscopic studies the gold particles are too small to be detected. The recent combination of the immunogold staining procedure in electron microscopy and the detection of gold particles in histological preparations by a silver precipitation reaction (Danscher, 1981), however, resulted in an extremely sensitive method, referred to as immunogold–silver staining (IGSS) (Holgate *et al.*, 1983). By this method the difficulty of immunostaining of regulatory peptides in nerves and endocrine cells in routinely fixed, paraffin-embedded material has been overcome (Hacker *et al.*, 1985).

Before applying immunocytochemical methods in light microscopy, tissues mostly undergo histological processing to preserve a good cellular detail. It can be postulated that an increasing preservation of the tissue structure concomitantly decreases immunoreactivity of many antigens. Hence, tissue fixation is the most critical factor in successful staining. For light-microscopic use, most of the immunocytochemical methods can be applied on paraffin sections of formalin-fixed tissue. A short fixation time is recommended, since prolonged exposure to fixatives may mask or destroy antigens. Sometimes pretreatment with proteolytic enzymes is necessary to unmask antigenic sites (Mepham *et al.*, 1979). One of the most preferable fixatives is a formaldehyde solution containing mercuric chloride (sublimate), which has to be removed before the staining procedure (Loeber *et al.*, 1983). Occasionally, special fixatives such as *p*-benzoquinone can prevent an unacceptable decrease in antigenicity by fixation as is the case for peptide neurotransmitters (Bishop *et al.*, 1978).

In ultrastructural immunocytochemistry especially, dehydration and plastic embedding procedures may destroy antigenic activity. Preembedding ultrastructural immunostaining, however, implies disadvantages, including often difficult penetration of antibodies into fresh or slightly fixed tissue slices together with poor preservation of the ultrastructural detail (Priestley, 1984). On the other hand, in postembedding immunocytochemistry, antigenicity is often lost. An important improvement is the development of cryoultramicrotomy, endeavoring to find a compromise between preservation of the ultrastructural detail and antigenic activity (Newman and Jasani, 1984).

3. *Qualitative and Quantitative Aspects*

One of the major problems for the pathologist is the detection of subtle changes. Species differences and aging must be taken into account. By randomizing and coding the slides of control and treated animals, however, readers' bias can be avoided. In immunocytochemistry semiquantitative reading is thus possible. The ascertainment of the average number and size of the immunoreactive cells and the intensity of the staining reaction will then be considered as a normal reaction serving as a baseline against which any change can be judged.

B. IMMUNOASSAYS

The effects of foreign compounds on the very dynamic endocrine system are often expressed as subtle changes in the levels of the circulating hormones. Such changes can be picked up by such sensitive methods as RIA. Since its discovery around 1960 by Yalow and Berson (1960) and by Elkins (1960), it has become almost a standard technique, which has been described in detail in several excellent textbooks (see e.g., Walker, 1977; Ekins, 1976; Abraham, 1977; Chard, 1978; Parker, 1981; Hunter and Corrie, 1983). In recent years this technique has been improved in several ways. First, several alternatives for the radiolabel have been described, including enzymes, fluorochromes, chemiluminescent probes, and metals, each of them having its own advantages and disadvantages with respect to cost, stability, and sensitivity (De Luca and McElroy, 1981; Weeks *et al.*, 1983; Woodhead *et al.*, 1981). Second, the discovery of the concept of monoclonal antibodies by Köhler and Milstein (1975) has opened the way to very specific assay systems. In addition, cloning makes available an infinite amount of each individual antibody, at least in theory, enabling the change to related techniques using multiple amounts of antibody compared to the original immunoassay (Weeks *et al.*, 1983; Woodhead *et al.*, 1981). Examples are the immunometric assays in which the antibody rather than the antigen is labeled, and the sandwich assays in which the antibody is coupled to a solid phase (Wood-

---

FIG. 2. Immunocytochemical staining (indirect peroxidase-labeled antibody method) for PRL, ACTH, TSH, LH, and FSH in the pituitary gland of adult untreated rats; ×300. PRL-immunoreactive cells are cup-shaped in female rats (a) and stellate with cytoplasmic processes lying between other cells in male rats (b); ACTH-positive cells are also stellate (c); TSH-producing cells are polygonal (d); FSH-immunoreactive cells (e) and round to polygonal LH-positive cells in a caudolateral area (f) show also weak or strong cytoplasmic staining.

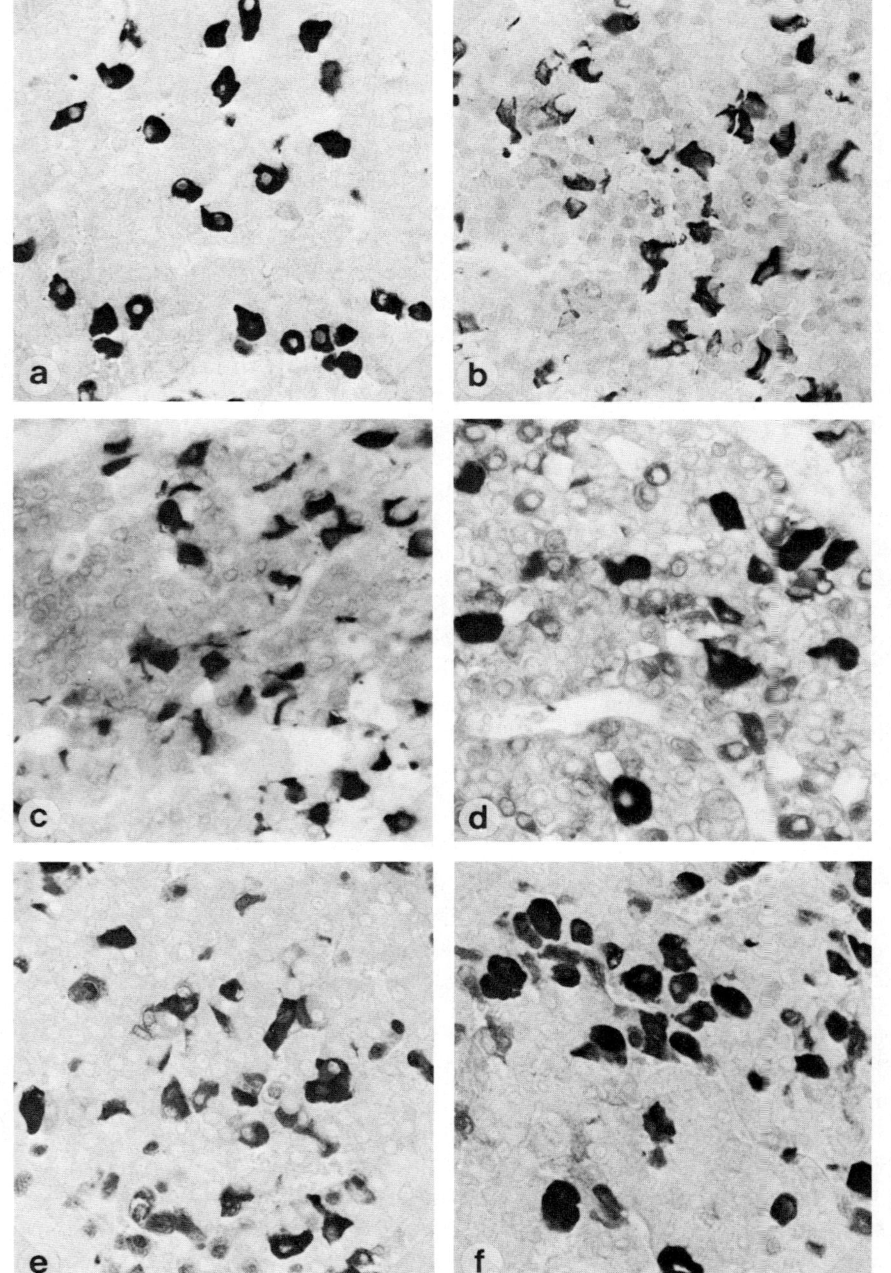
a
b
c
d
e
f

head *et al.*, 1974). Advantages of the immunometric assay are the lower detection limit and the rapidly obtained equilibrium leading to shorter assay procedures (Hunter and Budd, 1981). Nevertheless, the original RIA system will be used for at least another decade, if only for its simplicity and its favorable signal: noise ratio.

Scanning the literature will reveal that for virtually all endocrine parameters some sort of (radio)immunoassay has been developed. Consequently, there is a lively exchange of materials between investigators. Moreover, as stated before, a large number of reagents is available from the NIADDK in Bethesda, Maryland. For a number of nonspecific compounds (e.g., steroids, thyroid hormones) it is often also possible to turn to commercially available kits for their measurement in human specimens. Some modification may be necessary in order to decrease the required sample volume. In addition, attention has to be given to the fact that metabolism of steroids may differ between humans and laboratory animals, giving rise to unexpected cross-reacting metabolites.

Although in general both serum and plasma can be used in immunoassay procedures, there is a preference for serum due to the occurrence of coagulation during thawing of plasma samples. In certain cases urine may be the substrate of choice. Yet, it must be kept in mind that certain compounds (e.g., steroids) in urine are present as conjugates to glucuronic acid and sulfuric acid and, consequently, hydrolysis and/or extraction may be necessary (Abraham, 1977).

C. Function Tests

Function tests are a valuable tool in assessing the endocrine-toxic potential of chemical compounds. Due to the complexity of the endocrine system it is obvious that no single overall function test exists, but that each endocrine organ has its own specific test based upon the uptake of radioisotopes or its reaction to "externally" added hormonal stimuli.

In general, function tests are indicated when changes in weight or morphology of a particular organ and alterations in circulating hormone levels have been found. Various function tests will be described here.

For the anterior pituitary gland the function of the respective tropic hormone-producing cells can be examined by stimulation with hypothalamic releasing factors. By i.v. administration of LH-releasing hormone (LHRH or luliberin), the release of LH and FSH can be determined in the serum using RIA. In a similar manner thyrotropin-releasing hormone (TRH or thyroliberin) induces the secretion of TSH and PRL into the serum and CRH affects the ACTH-producing cells. At a given time interval after the i.v. injection, the animals can be decapitated and desanguinated for blood sampling, or in cannulated animals the sample can be taken via the cannula.

After ACTH administration the concentration of corticosterone can be determined in the serum as a measure of the adrenal cortex function. For the study of pancreas function, administration of glucose followed by the measurement of immunoreactive insulin (IRI) is most appropriate. With respect to this, it should be mentioned that oral administration of glucose produces higher insulin levels than parenteral administration, leading to equal hyperglycemia (McIntyre *et al.*, 1964).

In toxicological practice various release tests can be performed consecutively in cannulated animals. A procedure for this might be the following. Two to three days after insertion of the cannula the animals are fasted overnight and blood samples are taken before and 3, 5, 10, 15, and 20 min after i.v. injection of glucose (4 mmol/kg body weight) for IRI determination. Pituitary function can be tested in the same animals, 48 hr after the glucose tolerance test, with a 48- to 72-hr interval between the administration of TRH and LHRH (1 μg/kg body weight). For hormone determinations blood samples are taken before and 8, 20, and 60 min after administration of the releasing factor. For the various hormone concentrations in the serum of individual animals the area above the zero-time value is calculated and statistically evaluated. This method offers the advantage of the use of a small number of animals.

Besides the release tests, another type of function test is the uptake and release of radiolabel. For the assessment of thyroid function, for instance, the uptake of parenterally administered ^{125}I or ^{131}I (2 μCi/kg body weight) by the thyroid is well known. The radioactivity can be determined in excised thyroid glands, but it is also possible to anesthetize the animals and put them between the detectors of a γ counter. In this way individual rats can be screened for the uptake as well as release by determining the radioactivity 6, 24, and 48 (or 72) hr after administration of the radiolabel.

Also with noninvasive techniques function studies can be performed. The determination of 17-hydroxycorticosteroids in urine is an effective way to determine adrenocortical activity. An increase in 24-hr levels, whether or not after ACTH administration, regularly reflects hyperadrenocorticism. Furthermore, determination of suppression of corticosteroid production, by metyrapone, for instance, might be very useful.

D. Ectomy

An alternative procedure to study the involvement of particular endocrine organs in the onset of toxicological effects can be the removal (ectomy) of these organs (e.g., pituitary, gonads, adrenals). In addition to this, gonadectomy also provides a unique system to test the suppressive effects of hormonally active compounds on gonadotropin secretion by the hypothalamic–pituitary axis, since this control system is very sensitive to negative feedback effects (Foxcroft, 1983; Hess, 1983).

E. *In Vitro* Methods

After identification of an endocrine-toxic compound *in vivo,* application of *in vitro* test systems is potentially useful to establish the mechanism of action or the relative potency of chemical compounds to interfere with endocrine function. In principle every aspect of endocrine regulation tested *in vivo* can also be examined in cell or tissue culture, with the exception of feedback regulation. For this purpose uptake and release studies, the determination of the activity of enzymes involved in the biosynthesis or degradation of hormones, but in particular the determination of receptor-binding interactions can be used (Clark and Van Leeuwen, 1984). Toxic compounds can influence the binding characteristics of tropic hormones (of protein nature) with plasma membrane receptors (Tate *et al.,* 1975; Simonian *et al.,* 1982) or those of steroid hormones with receptors present in the cytosol or nuclei of cells (Clark and Peck, 1979; Gasson and Bourgeois, 1983). Binding of hormones to plasma membrane receptors is commonly associated with the stimulation of adenyl cyclase activity, resulting in an increase of intracellular cAMP. Binding to steroid receptors induces DNA replication and consequently protein synthesis. These biological responses of receptor binding should always be determined in conjunction with the effect of toxic compounds upon receptor-binding characteristics, since they are essential to enable the differentiation between an agonistic or an antagonistic effect.

V. Experimental Practice

A. Bromide

One of the earliest experiences in our institute with endocrine toxicology stems from routine tests to determine the toxicity of bromide ion. Bromide is a natural constituent of plants and animals and is therefore present in many food commodities. However, our interest was the additional exposure of humans to bromide as a result of the use of bromide-containing food additives, pesticides, and soil fumigants. Van Logten *et al.* (1974) showed that the most prominent effect of bromide ion toxicity in the rat was the impairment of the endocrine system. Besides growth retardation, changes in the relative weights of thyroid, adrenals, and prostate were found. These results were confirmed by a complex of histopathological changes. Primarily a remarkable activation of the thyroid gland was found, characterized by a reduction in follicle size accompanied by an increase in height of the follicular epithelium. In addition, a decrease in secretory activity of the prostate and impaired spermatogenesis was observed in males and a reduction in the number of corpora lutea in female rats. Both observations were suggestive of a diminished gonadotropin production by the pituitary gland. Furthermore, the adrenals showed a decreased vacuolization of the zona fasciculata, indicative of an increased corticosteroid release and/or decreased synthesis. It is obvious that as a consequence of the effects on the gonads, in a three-generation reproduction study with rats, a diminished fertility and even complete infertility was found (Van Leeuwen *et al.*, 1983).

The most striking and sensitive effect of bromide, however, was the effect on the thyroid gland. Therefore, attention was focused on the pituitary–thyroid axis. In order to investigate the effect of bromide on the thyroid, uptake experiments with radiolabeled iodide were carried out in animals fed a "chloride-free" diet. Restriction of sodium in the diet made it possible to achieve similar bromide levels in the circulation with a 10 times lower bromide load than needed for animals fed a normal diet (Rauws and Van Logten, 1975). It appeared that the effect on uptake and release of iodide was biphasic (Fig. 3). At the second highest dose, the uptake of iodide by the thyroid was enhanced, whereas at the highest dose this effect was less and the release seemed to be faster (Van Leeuwen *et al.*, 1983). This might be explained by an increased activation of the thyroid by TSH, whereas at the highest dose bromide-induced thyroid impairment is so large that even a stimulated thyroid is not able to take up enough iodide to fulfill the requirements. However, also a relatively diminished stimulatory activity of the pituitary at the highest dose cannot be excluded. Therefore, the involvement of the pituitary gland was further investigated by specific methods (Loeber *et al.*, 1983). Using RIA, thyroxine (T_4) levels in serum appeared to be decreased together with an increase in TSH. Histopathological examination revealed an activation of the thyroid (Fig. 4). With immunocytochemistry a decreased staining for T_4 in

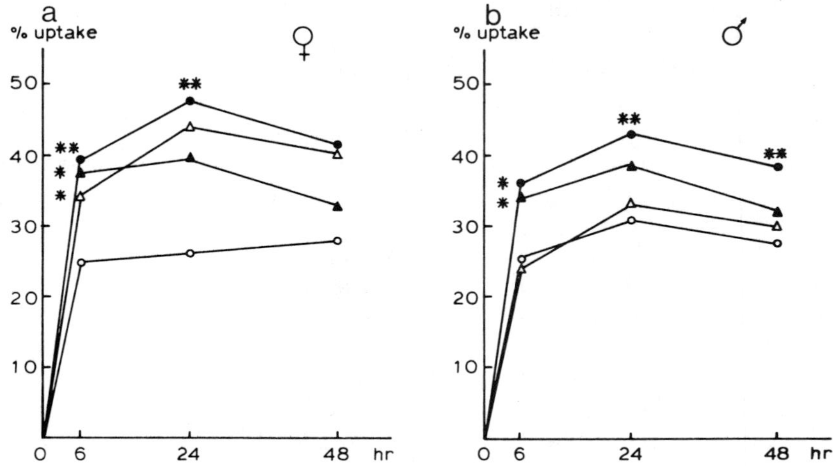

FIG. 3. Uptake of ^{131}I by the thyroid of female (a) and male (b) rats ($n = 8$) fed NaBr at dietary levels of 0 (control; ○), 125 (△), 500 (●), and 2000 (▲) mg/kg in a chloride-free diet for 90 days. Asterisks indicate values differing significantly from the corresponding control value: * $.01 \leq p < .05$; ** $0.001 \leq p < .01$.

the follicular epithelium and colloid in the thyroid gland was found in bromide-treated animals compared to controls (Fig. 5), whereas in the pituitary gland, TSH cells, revealed with anti-TSH serum, appeared to be more intensively stained in treated animals (Fig. 6). These effects predominantly point to a direct effect of bromide on the thyroid, leading to hypothyroidism with a consequent increase in stimulation of the pituitary gland due to feedback mechanisms. However, the observed increase in TSH is not sufficient to compensate for the decrease in serum T_4. Furthermore, function tests have shown that in bromide-treated animals the pituitary gland acts near its maximum capacity, since the increase in TSH after TRH administration is relatively small and of similar magnitude to that in control animals. Also in humans

---

FIG. 4. Thyroids of adult rats: (a) from control rat, with follicles lined by flat epithelium surrounding a lumen with colloid and (b) from rat fed 19,200 mg NaBr/kg diet for 4 weeks, strongly activated as judged from the heightening of the follicular epithelium and the decrease in amount and the more granular appearance of the colloid. Hematoxylin and eosin, ×300.

FIG. 5. Immunocytochemical staining (peroxidase–antiperoxidase antibody method) for thyroxin (T_4) in the thyroid of adult rats: (a) from control rat showing immunoreactivity in the colloid and in the follicular epithelium and (b) from rat fed 19,200 mg NaBr/kg diet for 4 weeks in which the follicles are less intensely strained. ×190.

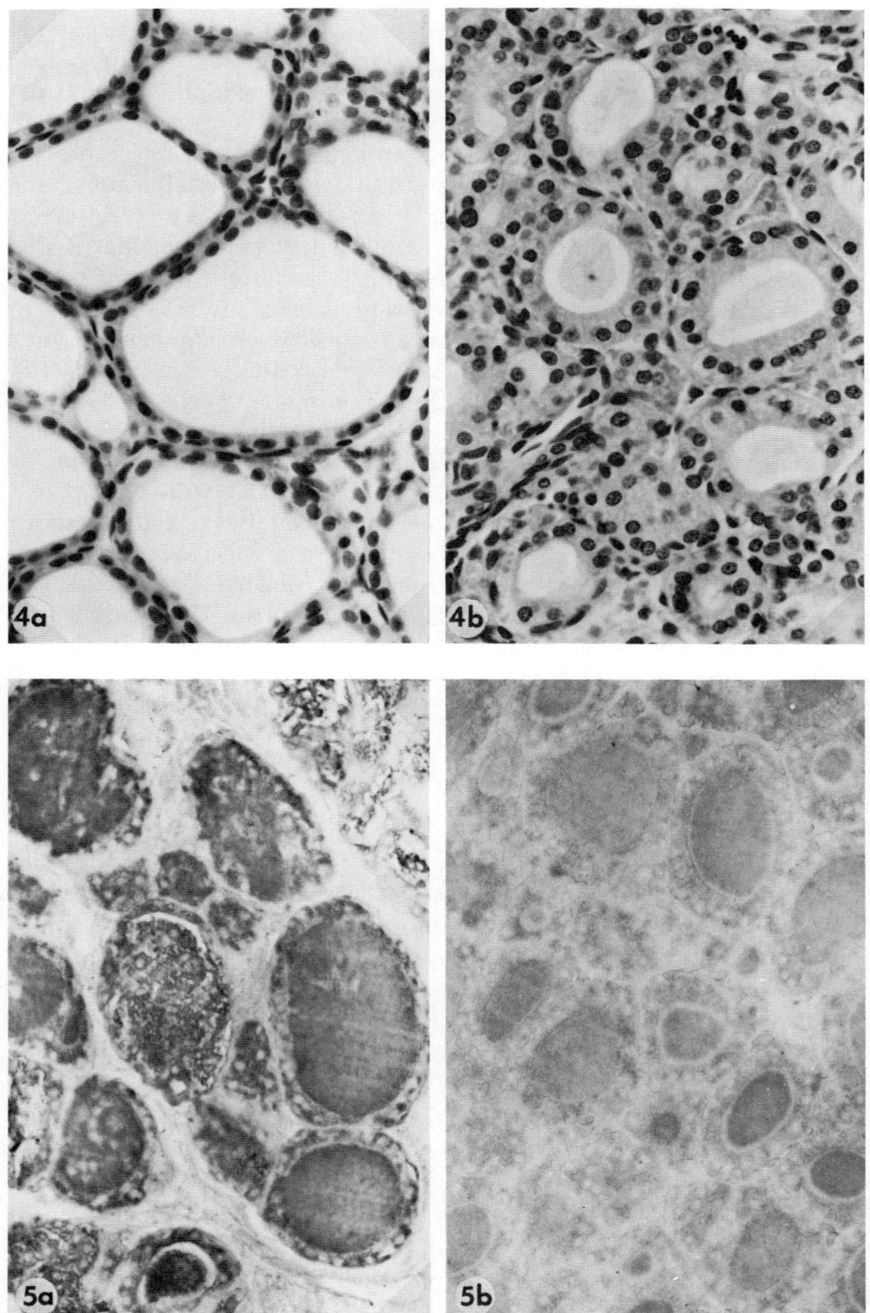
4a
4b
5a
5b

the thyroid gland is a target organ for bromide, although in a study with human volunteers, females showed a slight increase in the serum concentrations of thyroxine and triiodothyronine. which is in contrast to the observations in rats (Sangster *et al.*, 1983).

In addition, bromide also induced various other effects, like a decrease in serum testosterone, corticosterone, and growth hormone, and an increase in concentration of insulin and FSH (Loeber *et al.*, 1983). The latter is in accordance with the diminished spermatogenesis (Fig. 8), although it is puzzling that as a result of a deterioration of Leydig cells with a consequent fall in testosterone level, no rise in LH was found. For corticosterone, the bromide-induced decrease resulted via a feedback mechanism to an increased ACTH production, as assessed by an increase in immunoreactivity of ACTH-producing cells in the pituitary gland (Fig. 7). It can be concluded that histopathological and immunocytochemical findings correlate well with data on circulating hormones obtained by RIA. From these data it is postulated that bromide exerts a direct effect on thyroid and adrenal gland and possibly on the testes, leading via feedback regulation to increased tropic hormone stimulation. The effect on the testes, however, might also be mediated via a decrease in T_4, since it is known that T_4 stimulation is of importance for an adequate testicular function. At present, the underlying mechanism of bromide ion toxicity is still under investigation, and attention is focused upon the action of bromide ion on thyroid hormone biosynthesis.

B. TBTO

Another example of studies to explore the interaction of exogenous compounds with the endocrine system comprises short-term toxicity experiments with bis(tri-*n*-butyltin)oxide (TBTO) carried out in our institute by Krajnc *et al.* (1984). Besides strong immune effects, various endocrine alterations were found. The reduction in relative and absolute thyroid weight focused attention primarily on the pituitary–thyroid axis. Consistent with these weight changes, a decrease in con-

---

FIG. 6. Immunocytochemical staining (indirect peroxidase-labeled antibody method) for TSH in the pituitary gland of adult rats: (a) from control rat and (b) from rat fed 19,200 mg NaBr/kg diet for 12 weeks showing an increased number of strongly immunoreactive TSH cells. ×190.

FIG. 7. Immunocytochemical staining (indirect peroxidase-labeled antibody method) for ACTH in the pituitary gland of adult rats: (a) from control rat and (b) from rat fed 19,200 mg NaBr/kg diet for 12 weeks showing an increased number of strongly immunoreactive ACTH cells. ×190.

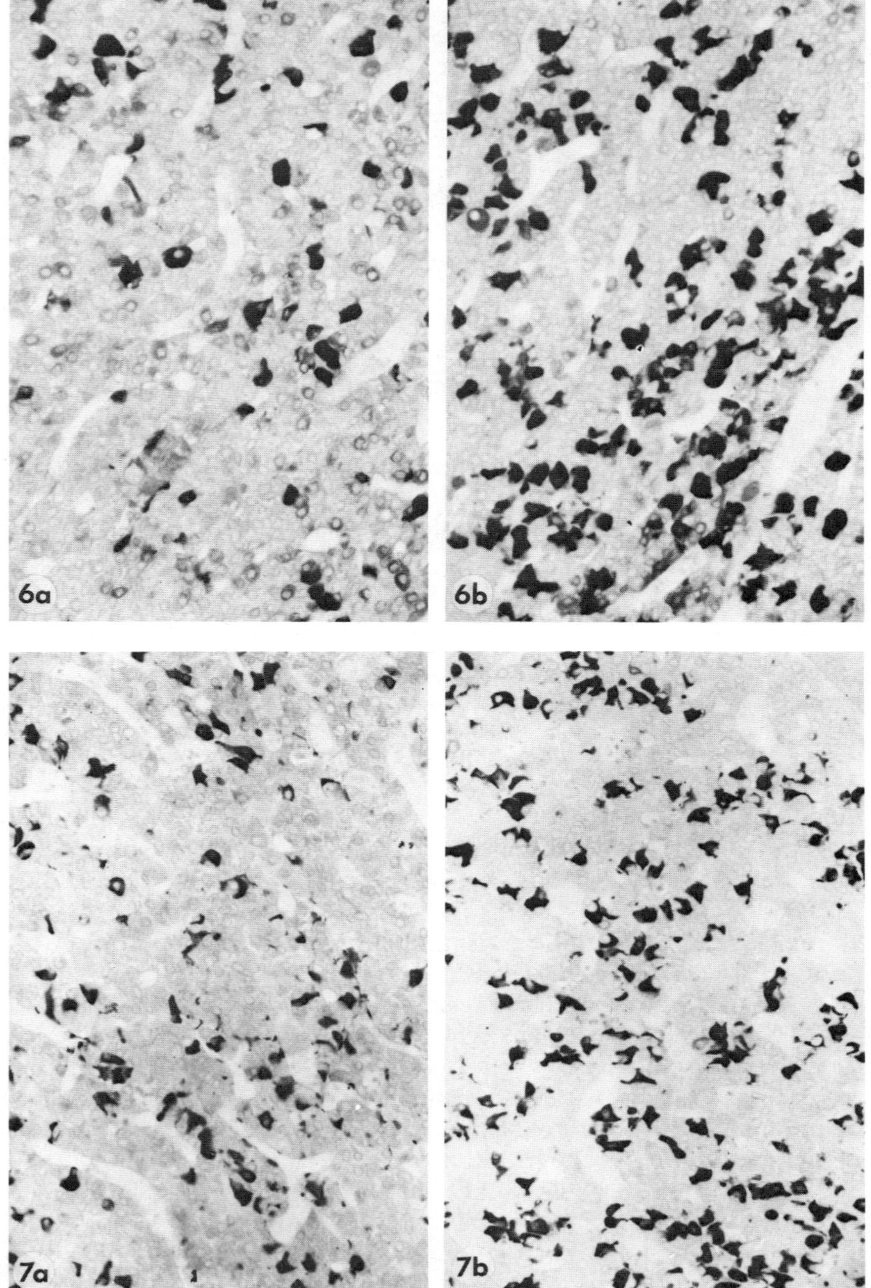

6a
6b
7a
7b

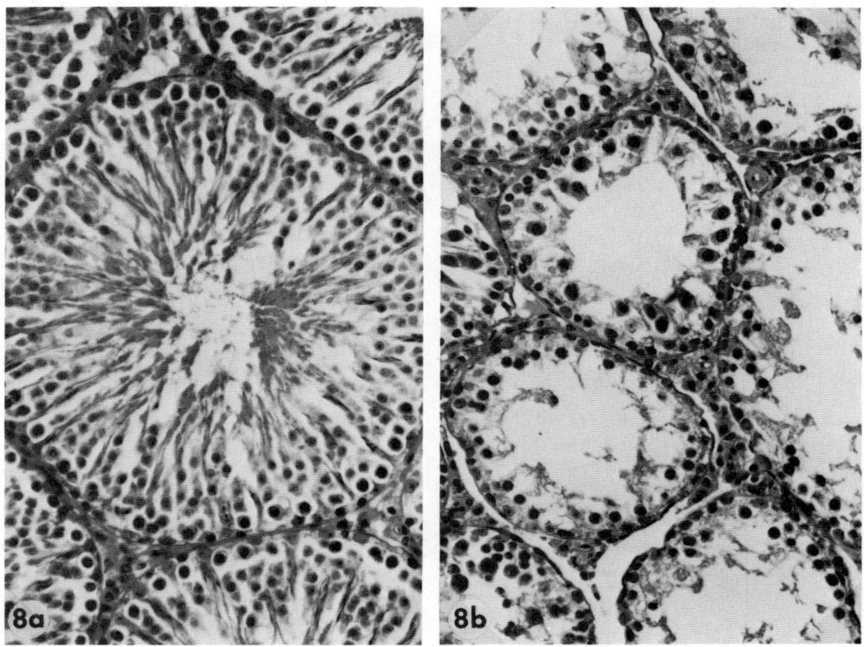

FIG. 8. Testes of adult rats: (a) from control rat and (b) from rat fed 19,200 mg NaBr/kg diet for 12 weeks showing decreased spermatogenesis and a reduction in diameter of the seminiferous tubules. Hematoxylin and eosin; ×190.

centration of T_4 and TSH in the serum was found. Morphologically, a flattening of epithelial cells of the thyroid indicating low activity was seen. In release studies the time course of TSH following TRH administration was changed, showing a diminished release in TBTO-treated animals (Fig. 9). In addition, immunohistochemical staining of the pituitary revealed a marked decrease in immunoreactivity for TSH (Fig. 10). All these observations correlate remarkably well and point to a TBTO-induced impairment of pituitary TSH production and secretion, resulting in a diminished thyroid gland function, as reflected by the decreased T_4 levels. This mechanism is contrary to that reported for bromide, where a thyroid hypofunction led to an increased stimulation of this organ via the pituitary by TSH.

Furthermore, TBTO also induced an increase in the concentration of LH in serum accompanied by the immunohistochemical finding of an increase in the number of LH-immunoreactive cells in the pituitary gland (Fig. 11). In accordance with these observations, LHRH admin-

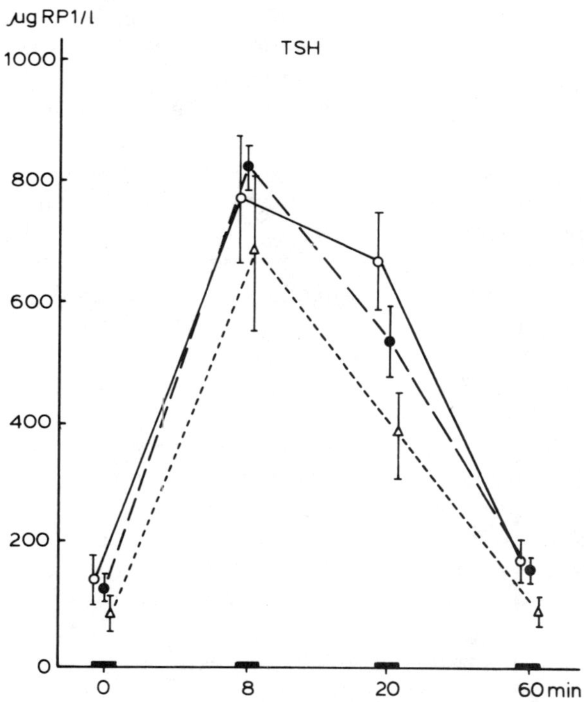

FIG. 9. Time course of serum TSH concentration in cannulated male rats in response to i.v.-administered thyrotropin-releasing hormone (1 µg TRH/kg body weight). Serial venous blood samples were drawn following 6 weeks of dietary TBTO exposure. Values (µg RP1/liter) are means of six to seven animals. Bars indicate ±1 SE. ○, Control; ●, 20 mg TBTO/kg feed; △, 80 mg TBTO/kg feed. [Reproduced from Krajnc *et al.* (1984), with permission.]

istration caused an increased LH release in TBTO-treated animals compared to controls. So, in contrast to the negative effect of TBTO on TSH-producing cells, there is a positive effect on LH production. No changes were found, however, in FSH concentration in the serum or in immunoreactivity of FSH-producing cells in the pituitary gland, although release tests showed a slightly increased capacity for FSH secretion.

C. β-HCH

In contrast to the above-mentioned compounds, the β isomer of hexachlorocyclohexane (β-HCH) probably is a compound exerting its effect on the endocrine system via a direct hormonal action. In the past β-HCH was present as a contaminant in technical formulations of the pesticide Lindane (γ-HCH). Due to its persistent nature, β-HCH is still present in the environment and consequently in the human food chain. In our institute experiments were carried out to determine the toxicity of β-HCH. In a subchronic toxicity study with rats, marked effects on the reproductive system have been observed comprising (1) reduced weight of the gonads; (2) atrophy of the testes, characterized by an atrophy of the seminiferous tubules, spermatogenic arrest, and a decrease in number of interstitial cells; (3) atrophy of the ovaries, with absence of corpora lutea; and (4) hyperplasia and metaplastic changes in the endometrial epithelium (Fig. 12) (Van Velsen *et al.,* 1986a). These effects were confirmed in other studies also revealing alterations in adrenal glands and accessory sex glands. Microscopically, hypertrophy of the zona fasciculata in the adrenal glands was found. Both the dorsolateral and the ventral prostate were atrophic, while the alveolar epithelium was hypertrophic. Histopathological alterations in seminal vesicles and coagulation glands were indicative of diminished function. As judged from the sections of vagina and uterus, all high-dose females appeared to be in estrus (Van Velsen *et al.,* 1986b). These changes all indicate an estrogenic action of β-HCH. Various other experiments have supported this hypothesis. In the classical bioassay for estrogenic activity using juvenile mice and rats, the uterotropic effect of β-HCH was confirmed (Loeber and Van Velsen, 1985). In rats the effects of β-HCH on lipid concentrations and lipoprotein pattern were similar to those of ethinyl estradiol (Van Giersbergen *et al.,* 1984). In studies with the life-bearing aquatic organism *Poecilia reticulata* (guppy), β-HCH induced (1) hypertrophy of the rough endoplasmic reticulum in the liver; (2) an increase in staining intensity of blood and of ascitic and interstitial tissue fluids; (3) hypertrophy of the endocardial lining macrophages due to hyalin droplets in lysosomes and accumulation of hyalin droplets in the kidney (Wester *et al.,* 1985). These observations are attributed to an excessive production of the yolk precursor vitellogenin, as assessed by slab-gel electrophoresis of

---

FIG. 10. Immunocytochemical staining (indirect peroxidase-labeled antibody method) for TSH in the pituitary gland of adult rats: (a) from control rat and (b) from rat fed 80 mg TBTO/kg diet for 6 weeks showing a marked reduction in number of strongly immunoreactive TSH cells. ×190.

FIG. 11. Immunocytochemical staining (indirect peroxidase-labeled antibody method) for LH in the pituitary gland of adult rats: (a) from control rat and (b) from rat fed 80 mg TBTO/kg diet for 6 weeks showing an increased number of strongly immunoreactive LH cells (pictures taken from the central part of the anterior lobe). ×190.

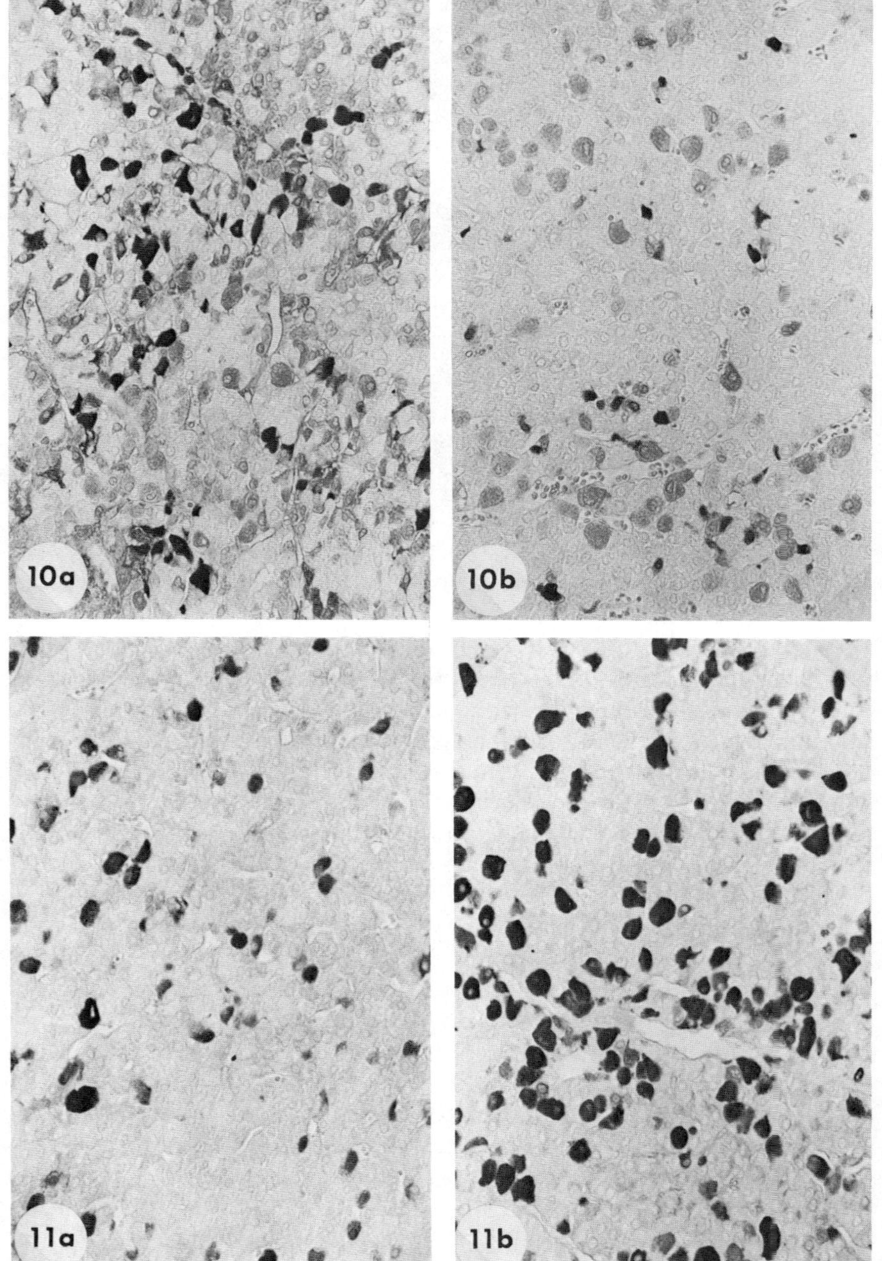
10a
10b
11a
11b

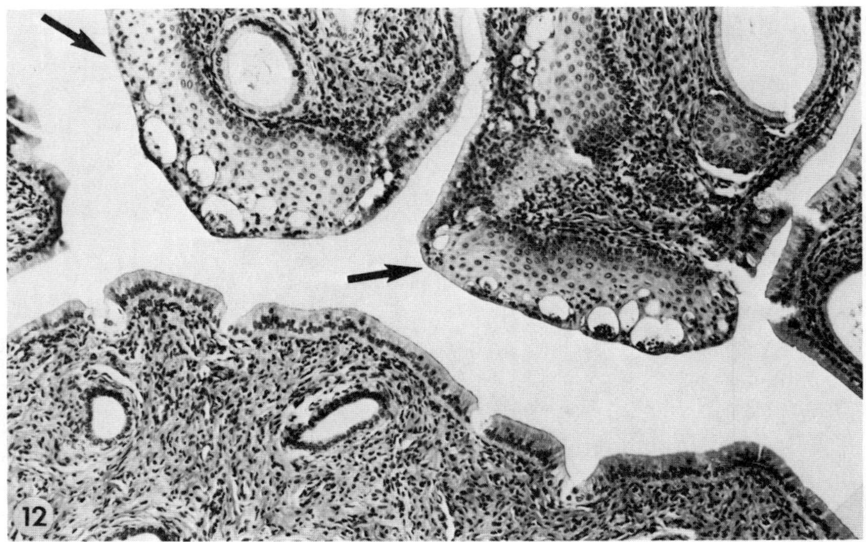

FIG. 12. Uterus of a rat fed 150 mg β-HCH/kg diet for 13 weeks showing endometrial epithelium indicative of estrus, and with focal metaplasia (arrows). Hematoxylin and eosin; ×95.

body fluids from juvenile male guppies. Similar morphological changes and an identical protein pattern were found when young fish were treated with 17β-estradiol. In the egg-laying Japanese ricefish (medaka, *Oryzias latipes*) β-HCH induced hermaphroditism in males and vitellogenesis in both sexes, characteristic of an estrogenic activity (Wester and Canton, 1986). Thus in mammalian as well as in nonmammalian species there is evidence for an estrogenic activity of β-HCH or its metabolites. To investigate the mechanism of action, *in vitro* experiments have been carried out with a human mammary tumor cell line (MCF-7) possessing estrogen receptors which are fully biologically active. In this system β-HCH induced the production of the progesterone receptor, which is regarded as the biological response of interaction with the estrogen receptor, although at the moment binding of β-HCH to the receptor itself could not be detected (Van Velsen and Coosen, 1986). Thus the mechanism of action of this estrogenic compound, having a saturated cycloalkane structure in contrast to the phenolic structure of the known estrogens, still has to be resolved.

In conclusion, it can be said that endocrine toxicology is a field of growing interest in routine toxicity testing. As was shown for bromide,

TBTO, and β-HCH, radiochemical findings, immunocytochemical observations, and the results of function tests correlate very well and offer a clear picture of the action of endocrine-toxic substances. In addition to *in vivo* information, *in vitro* tests can be very helpful in resolving the mechanism of action.

References

Abraham, G. E. (1977). "Handbook of Radioimmunoassays." Dekker, New York.

Andrews, W. W., and Ojeda, S. R. (1981). *Endocrinology* **109,** 2032–2039.

Barrett, A. M., and Stockham, M. A. (1963). *J. Endocrinol.* **26,** 97–105.

Berchtold, J. P. (1977). *Histochemistry* **50,** 175–190.

Bishop, A. E., Pollak, J. M., Bloom, S. R., and Pearse, A. G. E. (1978). *J. Endocrinol.* **77,** 25–26.

Chard, T. (1978). "An Introduction to Radioimmunoassays and Related Techniques." North-Holland Publ., Amsterdam.

Clark, J. H., and Peck, E. J. (1979). "Monographs in Endocrinology." Springer-Verlag, New York.

Clark, J. H., and Van Leeuwen, F. X. R. (1984). Evaluation of short-term tests for non-genotoxic effects; Scientific Group on Methodologies for Safety Evaluation of Chemicals (SGOMSEC), Ottawa.

Cupps, T. R., and Fauci, A. S. (1982). *Immunol. Rev.* **65,** 133–155.

Danscher, G. (1981). *Histochemistry* **71,** 81–88.

De Luca, M., and McElroy, W. D., eds. (1981). Academic Press, London.

Döhler, K. D., and Wuttke, W. (1976). *Acta Endocrinol.* **83,** 269–279.

Döhler, K. D., Gärtner, K., Mühlen, A., von zur, and Döhler, H. (1977). *Acta Endocrinol.* **86,** 489.

Ekins, R. P. (1960). *Clin. Chim. Acta* **5,** 453.

Ekins, R. P. (1976). *In* "Hormone Assays and their Clinical Application" (J. A. Lorraine and E. T. Bell, eds.), 4th Ed., p. 1. Churchill-Livingstone, Edinburgh/London.

Faulk, W. P., and Taylor, G. M. (1971). *Immunochemistry* **8,** 1081–1083.

Foxcroft, G. R. (1983). O.I.E. Symposium on Sanitary Aspects Concerning the Control and Use of Anabolics in Animal Production, Paris.

Foxcroft, G. R., and Hess, D. L. (1986). *In* "Drug Residues in Animals" (A. G. Rico, ed.), pp. 147–174. Academic Press, Orlando, Florida.

Gasson, J. C., and Bourgeois, S. (1983). *UCLA Symp. Mol. Cell. Biol.* pp. 153–176.

Geuze, H. J., Slot, J. W., Van der Ley, P. A., and Scheffer, R. C. T. (1981). *J. Cell Biol.* **89,** 653–665.

Graham, R. C., Jr., and Karnovsky, M. J. (1966). *J. Histochem. Cytochem.* **14,** 291–302.

Guyton, A. C. (1976). "Textbook of Medical Physiology." Saunders, Philadelphia.

Hacker, G. W., Springall, D. R., Van Noorden, S., Bishop, A. E., Grimelius, L., and Polak, J. M. (1985). *Virchows Arch. Pathol. Anat.* **406,** 449–461.

Harwood, E. J. (1982). *Lab. Anim.* **16,** 314–318.

Hess, D. L. (1983). O.I.E. Symposium on Sanitary Aspects Concerning the Control and Use of Anabolics in Animal Production, Paris.

Holgate, C. S., Jackson, P., Cowen, P. N., and Bird, C. C. (1983). *J. Histochem Cytochem.* **31,** 938–944.

Hsu, S. M., Raine, L., and Fangen, H. (1981). *J. Histochem. Cytochem.* **29,** 577–580.

Hunter, W. M., and Budd, P. S. (1981). *J. Immunol. Methods* **45,** 255–273.

Hunter, W. M., and Corrie, J. E. T. (1983). "Immunoassays for Clinical Chemistry." Churchill Livingstone, Edinburgh.
IARC (1979). "Monographs on the Evaluation of the Carcinogenic Risk of Chemicals to Humans." Sex Hormones (II), Vol. 21.
Köhler, G., and Milstein, C. (1975). *Nature (London)* **256,** 495.
Krajnc, E. I., Wester, P. W., Loeber, J. G., Van Leeuwen, F. X. R., Vos, J. G., Vaessen, H. A. M. G., and Van der Heijden, C. A. (1984). *Toxicol. Appl. Pharmacol.* **75,** 363–386.
Krulich, L., Hefco, E., Illner, P., and Read, C. B. (1974). *Neuroendocrinology* **16,** 293.
Lawson, N., Jenning, R. J., Pollard, A. D., Shirten, R. G., Ralph, S. J., Marsden, C. A., Fears, R., and Brindley, P. N. (1981). *Biochem. J.* **200,** 265–273.
Liener, I. (1979). *J. Am. Oil Chem.* **56,** 121–129.
Loeber, J. G., and Van Velsen, F. L. (1985). *Food Addit. Contam.* **1,** 63–66.
Loeber, J. G., Franken, M. A. M., and Van Leeuwen, F. X. R. (1983). *Food Chem. Toxicol.* **21,** 391–404.
Luster, M. I., Pfeifer, R. W., and Tucker, A. N. (1985) *In* "Endocrine Toxicology" (J. A. Thomas, K. S. Korach, and J. A. McLachlan, eds.), pp. 67–83. Raven, New York.
McIntyre, N., Holdsworth, C. D., and Turner, D. S. (1964). *Lancet* **2,** 20–21.
Maji, T., Yoshida, A., and Ashida, K. (1980). *Nutr. Rep. Int.* **21,** 437–445.
Mattheij, J. A. M., and van Pijkeren, T. A. (1984). *Acta Endocrinol.* **84,** 51–61.
Mepham, B. L., Fraten, W., and Mitchell, B. S. (1979). *Histochem. J.* **11,** 345–357.
Nakane, P. K., and Pierce, J. B., Jr. (1966). *J. Histochem. Cytochem.* **14,** 929–931.
Newman, G. R., and Jasani, B. (1984). *In* "Immunolabelling for Electron Microscopy" (J. M. Polak and I. M. Varndell, eds.), pp. 53–70. Elsevier, Amsterdam.
Parekh, C. K., and Coulston, F. (1983). O.I.E. Symposium on Sanitary Aspects Concerning the Control and Use of Anabolics in Animal Production, Paris.
Parker, C. W. (1981). *Annu. Rev. Pharmacol. Toxicol.* **21,** 113.
Priestley, J. V. (1984). *In* "Immunolabelling for Electron Microscopy" (J. M. Polak and I. M. Varndell, eds.), pp. 37–52. Elsevier, Amsterdam.
Rackis, J. J. (1974). *J. Am. Oil Chem. Soc.* **51,** 161A–174A.
Rauws, A. G., and Van Logten, M. J. (1975). *Toxicology* **3,** 29–32.
Romano, E. L., and Romano, M. (1977). *Immunochemistry* **14,** 711–715.
Sangster, B., Blom, J. L., Sekhuis, V. M., Loeber, J. G., Rauws, A. G., and Koedam, J. C. (1983). *Food Chem. Toxicol.* **21,** 409–419.
Shivanandappa, T., and Krishnakumari, M. K. (1983). *Acta Pharmacol. Toxicol.* **52,** 12–17.
Simonian, M. H., White, M. L., and Gill, G. N. (1982). *Endocrinology* **111,** 919.
Singh, D. V., Anderson, R. R., and Turner, C. W. (1971). *J. Endocrinol.* **50,** 445–450.
Steffens, A. B. (1969). *Physiol. Behav.* **4,** 833.
Sternberger, L. A. (1979). "Immunochemistry," pp. 104–169. Wiley, New York.
Straus, W. (1982). *J. Histochem. Cytochem.* **30,** 491–493.
Tate, R. L., Schwarz, H. I., Holmers, J. M., Kohn, L. D., and Winand, R. J. (1975). *J. Biol. Chem.* **250,** 6509.
Van Giersbergen, P. L. M., Danse, L. H. J. C., Van Velsen, F. L., and Van Leeuwen, F. X. R. (1984). *Med. Fac. Landbouww. Gent* **49/3b,** 1195–1202.
Van Leeuwen, F. X. R., Den Tonkelaar, E. M., and Van Logten, M. J. (1983). *Food Chem. Toxicol.* **21,** 383–389.
Van Logten, M. J., Wolthuis, M., Rauws, A. G., Kroes, R. Den Tonkelaar, E. M., Berkvens, H., and Van Esch, G. J. (1974). *Toxicology* **2,** 257–267.
Van Velsen, F. L., and Coosen, R. (1986). *Toxicol. Appl. Pharmacol.* (submitted).

Van Velsen, F. L., Danse, L. H. J. C., Van Leeuwen, F. X. R., Dormans, J. A. M., and Van Logten, M. J. (1986a). *Fundam. Appl. Toxicol.* **6,** 697–712.

Van Velsen, F. L., Franken, M. A. M. and Loeber, J. G. (1986b). *Toxicol. Appl. Pharmacol.* (submitted).

Vos, J. G. (1977). *CRC Crit. Rev. Toxicol.* **5,** 67–101.

Walker, W. H. C. (1977). *Clin. Chem.* **23,** 384.

Weeks, I., McCapra, F., Campbell, A. K., and Woodhead, J. S. (1983). *In* "Immunoassays for Clinical Chemistry" (W. M. Hunter and J. E. T. Corrie, eds.), p. 525. Churchill Livingstone, Edinburgh.

Wester, P. W., and Canton, J. H. (1986). *Aquat. Toxicol.* **9,** 21–45.

Wester, P. W., Canton, J. H., and Bisschop, A. (1985). *Aquat. Toxicol.* **6,** 271–296.

Wisser, H., and Breuer, H. (1981). *J. Clin. Chem. Clin. Biochem.* **19,** 323–337.

Woodhead, J. S., Addison, G. M., and Hales, C. N. (1974). *Br. Med. Bull.* **30,** 44–49.

Woodhead, J. S., Simpson, J. S. A., Weeks, I., Patel, A., Campbell, A. K. Hart, R., Richardson, A., and McCapra, F. (1981). *In* "Monoclonal Antibodies and Developments in Immunoassay" (A. Albertine and R. Ekins, eds.), pp. 135–145. Elsevier, Amsterdam.

Yalow, R. S., and Berson, S. A. (1960). *J. Clin. Invest.* **39,** 1157.

Uses of γ-Glutamyltransferase in Experimental Toxicology

J. P. BRAUN,* G. SIEST,† AND A. G. RICO*

**Laboratoire Associé INRA de Toxicologie Biochimique et Métabolique, Ecole Nationale Vétérinaire, F-31076 Toulouse Cedex, France*

†Laboratoire de Biochimie Pharmacologique, Faculté des Sciences Pharmaceutiques et Biologiques, F-54000 Nancy, France

I. Introduction

γ-Glutamyltransferase (GGT, E.C. 2.3.2.2) has been widely investigated for the last 20 years, and its diagnostic uses in humans as well as in animals have been extensively reviewed (Schmidt and Schmidt, 1973; Rosalki, 1975; Braun *et al.*, 1977; Goldberg, 1980; Siest and Heusghem, 1982).

GGT is a membrane-bound glycoprotein which catalyzes the first step of glutathione breakdown. Structural studies were mainly focused on kidney GGT, which is a dimer composed of two nonidentical subunits: the larger one (MW 51×10^3) contains a short hydrophobic NH_2-terminal segment anchoring the protein into the membrane, whereas the lighter subunit supports the catalytic site. Sialylation of the enzyme is highly variable.

The physiological role and interest of this enzyme are growing each year. Among its many functions are the transfer of amino acids across cell membranes, the regulation of glutathione breakdown and glutathione conjugation, and the metabolism of eicosanoids.

In experimental toxicology, liver GGT is not an index of cell damage. Due to its cellular localization, however, it is now widely used in two main fields: hepatic pharmacological induction and chemical liver carcinogenesis. In contrast, kidney GGT is an index of cell damage used in toxicity testing.

II. Distribution of the Enzyme

A. Distribution in the Organs of the Animals

In all adult mammals and birds, GGT is mainly in the kidneys in which its catalytic concentration differs according to species and age as shown in Table I; kidney GGT levels are highest in rodents, which exhibit a very low liver GGT activity. Moreover, kidney GGT concentration is significantly higher in male than in female rats (Braun *et al.,* 1978b; Jedrzejewski and Kugler, 1982), mice (Braun *et al.,* 1978a), and guinea pigs (Sobiech and Szewczuk, 1974). Such a difference was demonstrated to be testosterone-dependent, as kidney GGT was lower in castrated male rats and could be compensated by testosterone (Malyusz and Ehrens, 1983).

Some species have a very low level of liver GGT (e.g., birds, cats, dogs, rats, mice), whereas other species have a relatively high liver GGT activity ranging from 5 to 58% of kidney cortex activity. Moreover, moderately high GGT concentrations are also observed in the pancreas, mammary gland, and intestine, along which the activity decreases from the jejunum to the ileum in the dog (Levanti *et al.,* 1978).

Changes in GGT concentration with age have been reported. In the fetus and newborn mice and rats, liver GGT is relatively elevated and highly glycosylated; then it decreases dramatically and remains low for all the rest of the life (Braun *et al.,* 1978a; Igarashi *et al.,* 1981; Fujiwara *et al.,* 1982), except in liver tumors (see Section IV). On the contrary, in mice (Braun *et al.,* 1978a), rats (Wapnir *et al.,* 1982), pigs (Collis and Stark, 1977), and rabbits (Sassowa, 1968), kidney GGT is low at birth and increases steadily for the first weeks of life, remaining stable thereafter.

B. Cellular and Subcellular Distribution

Within the organs, GGT is not homogeneously distributed. For instance, in the liver it is mainly located in the epithelia of bile ducts and at the biliary pole of the hepatocytes; in adult rat liver on which most induction and cancerogenesis experiments are carried out, GGT was also demonstrated in Kupffer and other nonparenchymal cells (Siest *et*

TABLE I

PERCENTAGE DISTRIBUTION OF γ-GLUTAMYLTRANSFERASE IN THE ORGANS OF SOME SPECIES OF MAMMALS[a]

Species	Number of animals	Kidney	Liver	Pancreas	Spleen	Intestine	Muscle	Brain	References
Horse	10	100	20	17	ND	2	1	1	Ford and Adam (1981)
Cow	10	100	8	37	1	1	1	ND	Rico *et al.* (1977)
Ewe	10	100	9	8	2	1	1	ND	Braun *et al.* (1977)
Goat	—	100	14	ND	ND	ND	2	ND	Majumder and Ganguli (1972)
Swine	10	100	16	52	17	9	1	ND	Rico *et al.* (1977)
Dog	6	100	1	122	1	27	1	ND	Keller (1981)
Rat	—	100	4	ND	12	ND	1	ND	Szasz (1974)
Mouse	—	100	1	13	50	1	1	1	Findeisen (1972)
Guinea pig	—	100	2	42	5	1	1	1	Findeisen (1972)
Rabbit	—	100	1	2	1	1	0	ND	Findeisern (1972)
Hamster	—	100	1	52	ND	ND	ND	ND	Albert *et al.* (1964)
Baboon	8	100	5	80	3	3	1	ND	Braun *et al.* (1980)
Macaque	10	100	4	47	2	2	1	ND	Braun *et al.* (1980)

[a]Results are given as percentage of kidney cortex activity concentration which cannot be compared because of differences in analytical procedures. ND, No data.

al., 1982a); in neonatal rat liver a high enzyme activity was observed throughout the hepatic lobule with some predominance in the periportal area (Müller *et al.,* 1974; Kitagawa *et al.,* 1980a). In the pancreas, there is no GGT in Langerhans islets; in the kidney, GGT concentration is much higher in the brush border of proximal tubules than in the rest of the nephron (Heinle *et al.,* 1977; Shimada *et al.,* 1982).

In early experiments, GGT was separated by centrifugation with the "microsomal" fraction; it was then shown that the activity was mainly bound to the plasma membrane and other cell membranes, whereas the free "soluble" form of the enzyme was not usually higher than 10% of total cell activity.

In the membranes, GGT is at the outside surface and can be released in the cytosol or the external medium by different reagents and drugs; but for complete solubilization, it requires the use of detergents or of proteases (Siest *et al.,* 1982a).

C. GGT in Body Fluids

Serum or plasma GGT have been separated into various molecular forms which are not true isoenzymes and the significance of which remains to be discussed (Artur *et al.,* 1984). Plasma GGT originates from liver and perhaps pancreas (Gibinski and Aleksandrowitch, 1965; Naftalin *et al.,* 1969), and its activity is normally moderate or low in most animal species or humans; it is even very low in cats, dogs, rats, mice, and birds (Braun *et al.,* 1982).

Urine GGT originates only from the kidney in humans as well as in mammals; it has the same electrophoretic and immunological patterns as the kidney enzyme (Kuska and Kokot, 1970; Scherberich and Gauhl, 1978; Scherberich *et al.,* 1978).

High GGT concentrations were also found in bile, colostrum, milk, and pancreatic and seminal fluids. Moderate activities have been reported in peritoneal and synovial fluids, but no activity could be measured in cerebrospinal fluid (Braun *et al.,* 1977).

III. Hepatic Induction and Hepatic Disturbances

A. Toxic Disturbances of the Liver

Usually, hepatocyte damage (e.g., by CCl_4) is responsible only for a moderate or no elevation of serum or plasma GGT: it was shown to be increased twofold in ponies dosed with 0.5 ml CCl_4/kg (Noonan, 1981), rabbits (Sledzinski and Kokot, 1977), horses (Ikeda *et al.*, 1976), and rats (Ideo *et al.*, 1972).

On the contrary, plasma GGT activity was shown to be dramatically increased in experimental bile duct ligation and in sporidesmin-induced cholestasis (Ford, 1974; Towers and Smith, 1978; Towers and Stratton, 1978; Bézille *et al.*, 1984). Sporidesmin is a mycotoxin originating from *Pithomyces chartarum;* it produces a very severe cholangitis and pericholangitis resulting in intrahepatic cholestasis and eventually in cirrhosis. Impaired liver metabolism of chlorophyll is responsible for an accumulation of phylloerythrin in the skin and a secondary photosensitization, that is, facial eczema, which is the only apparent sign of the disease. In clinically ill ewes, plasma GGT can be higher than 1000 units/liter (normal < 80 units/liter) (Bézille *et al.*, 1984), and it is considered the best indicative test of liver damage in sporidesmin toxicity (Towers and Stratton, 1978).

Other toxic injuries to the liver were also demonstrated to elevate serum GGT: *Amanita phalloides* or phalloidin intoxication of rabbits (Palyza *et al.*, 1969) and dogs (Floersheim *et al.*, 1978); in rats acetylaminofluorene (AAF)-transformed liver cells were less sensitive to phalloidin than GGT-negative cells (Sawada *et al.*, 1982). In experimental lupinosis of sheep, GGT increases were correlated with degeneration and necrosis of hepatocytes (Malherbe *et al.*, 1977); in tetrodotoxin intoxication of rats, serum GGT increased as chronic hepatitis developed (Roushdy and Mansour, 1980).

B. Liver Drug Induction

It has been long known that increases of plasma GGT can be induced by numerous drugs, chemicals, and ethanol. Alcohol-related changes of GGT have been covered extensively elsewhere (Rosalki, 1974, 1977; Lamy *et al*, 1975; Braun and Fernet, 1982) and will not be discussed here.

When discussing the induction of liver GGT, two different topics have to be considered separately: (1) increases of GGT within the liver and (2) possible increases of plasma GGT which can be very moderate or even not observed.

1. Induction of Liver GGT

Most experiments have dealt with rodents after phenobarbital (PB) treatment was demonstrated to increase liver GGT in the rat (Ideo *et al.*, 1971). PB induces diffuse elevations of GGT, some of them in ductular proliferations, primarily in part 1 (periportal) of the liver acinus; but PB, unlike carcinogens, does not induce GGT-positive foci (Capouya and Lindahl, 1983; Moore *et al.*, 1983a; Schwarz *et al.*, 1983). The inducing effects of such compounds as PB or ethanol are only transient, and GGT activity decreases regularly after their withdrawal. Moreover, PB can also enhance the neoplastic progression of chemically induced liver cancers in the rat; in such occurrences GGT is observed in foci and does not decrease after the withdrawal of PB (see Section IV).

In rat liver, PB treatment (50 mg/kg twice a day for 5 days) induced significant increases of total liver GGT, but the effects were more intense in nonparenchymal cells than in hepatocytes (Galteau *et al.*, 1980). Moreover, in PB-treated rats and rabbits, GGT was much more enhanced in plasma membranes than in other liver fractions. Therefore, experiments dealing with drug-induced variations of GGT should check GGT in the total homogenate and in plasma membranes as well as other cell fractions.

Other compounds have also been shown to have such inducing effects on liver GGT:

1. In the rat: aflatoxin B_1 (AFB_1) (Kamden *et al.*, 1981, 1982), hexachlorobenzene (Adjarov *et al.*, 1982), halothane (Lavinski, 1968), stilbestrol (Szacki and Lawinski, 1969), aminopyrine (Igarashi *et al.*, 1982), 4-aminoantipyrine (Satoh *et al.*, 1982), 1-naphthylisothiocyanate (Richards *et al.*, 1982b), DDT, and toxaphene (Garcia and Mourelle, 1984), but neither methylcholanthrene (MC), Aroclor (Garthoff *et al.*, 1981), 4-acetamidoantipyrine (Satoh *et al.*, 1982), nor pregnenolone-16-carbonitrile (PAC) (Siest *et al.*, 1982b)
2. In the mouse: Aroclor (Siest *et al.*, 1982b) but not MC, β-naphthoflavone, or PAC (Siest *et al.*, 1982b)
3. In the rabbit: Hexachlorophene (Ivanov *et al.*, 1976) but not β-naphthoflavone or PAC (Bagrel *et al.*, 1980)
4. In the guinea pig: PB (Siest *et al.*, 1982b)
5. In the dog: prednisone (Badylak and Van Vleet, 1982)

The response to PB was higher in the rabbit than in the rat, in which it was more intense than in the guinea pig (Roomi and Goldberg, 1981).

But the comparative results should be examined cautiously: the elevation of GGT is time-dependent and the precise time course for each inducer in each species has to be defined. The induction is also dose-dependent.

Moreover, liver GGT was also shown to be increased in aging Donryu rats, in which it was gradually elevated from the thirtieth week of life. At the ninetieth week, liver GGT was about 20 times as high as in young adults but still only 40% of that of fetal liver; the elevation of GGT was mainly located in the periportal hepatocytes (Kitagawa *et al.*, 1980b). In Wistar and Fischer 344 old rats, GGT-positive foci could also be observed and were similar to those of the early stages of chemical carcinogenesis (Ogawa *et al.*, 1981), although no visible hyperplastic nodule could be observed.

After portocaval shunt in rats, GGT was first increased around the lobule, then it spread toward the center of the lobule (Müller *et al.*, 1974). Portocaval shunt is also responsible for a functional deficiency of the liver which reduces chemically induced tumors by such procarcinogens as 3′-methyl dimethylamino azobenzene which requires hepatic activation (Fiala *et al.*, 1978).

Following partial hepatectomy, rat liver GGT was not increased (Fiala and Fiala, 1973; Cameron *et al.*, 1978; Schultz-Ellinson *et al.*, 1981).

In cell cultures, adult rat hepatocytes showed characteristics of fetal liver and their GGT content was increased from the sixth day of culture; such an elevation was delayed and lowered by glucocorticoids (Colombo and Gigon, 1979; Colona *et al.*, 1981).

2. *Increases of Serum GGT*

In rats and rabbits, the induction of liver GGT was not consistently associated with an elevation of plasma GGT (Bagrel *et al.*, 1980), although an 18-day treatment of rabbits with PB induced twofold increase of plasma GGT (Ratanasavahn *et al.*, 1981). In PB-treated rabbits and guinea pigs but not in rats, plasma GGT was correlated with liver GGT (Huseby, 1979; Goldberg *et al.*, 1981; Roomi and Goldberg, 1981). GGT was more easily removed from plasma membrane and microsomes of the liver of PB-treated rabbits than from the liver of controls; the longer the duration of PB treatment, the more liver GGT could be solubilized by bile salts (Tazi *et al.*, 1980; Ratanasavahn *et al.*, 1982) but not by proteases such as bromelain or papain (Ratanasavahn *et al.*, 1984). Such an effect could be accounted for by PB-induced changes of membrane lipid composition (Ratanasavahn *et al.*, 1981).

In dogs, plasma GGT was not elevated by diphenylhydantoin or primidone treatments (Meyer and Noonan, 1981), but it was increased by dexamethasone (De Novo and Prasse, 1983), methylprednisolone (Meyer, 1982), and prednisone (Badylak and Van Vleet, 1982).

Following partial hepatectomy in rats, serum GGT showed a peak increase at the sixth hour and returned to normal on the twenty-fourth (Sekas and Cook, 1979).

IV. GGT and Experimental Carcinogenesis

A. Variations of Liver GGT with Carcinogenesis

As early as 1969, Fiala and Fiala showed that GGT activity was increased in microsomal preparations obtained from rat hepatomas induced by 3′-methyl-4-(dimethylamino)benzene and also from Novikoff and Morris 5123A hepatomas. Liver GGT has now become a widely used marker of early changes in liver carcinogenesis resulting from exposure to chemicals or from the transformation of cells in culture.

Since that time, similar increases of GGT were observed in the following situations:

1. Chemically induced tumors: AFB_1 (Zawirska, 1982; Appleton and Campbell, 1983), dimethylnitrosamine (DMN) (Fiala and Fiala, 1971; Fiala *et al.,* 1976; Tsuchida *et al.,* 1979), diethylnitrosamine (DEN) (Pitot *et al.,* 1978; Ford and Pereira, 1980; Tatematsu *et al.,* 1980; Yager and Yager, 1980; Kojima *et al.,* 1981; Milks *et al.,* 1982; Stout and Becker, 1982; Pereira *et al.,* 1984; Sirica *et al.,* 1984; Tsuda *et al.,* 1984), azaserine (Takahashi *et al.,* 1979), dimethylbenzanthracene (DMBA) (Onoé *et al.,* 1976; Pereira *et al.,* 1983), Dimethylhydrazine (DMH) (Fiala *et al.,* 1977; Columbano *et al.,* 1982; Ying *et al.,* 1982; Pereira *et al.,* 1983), 1,2-dibromoethane, benzopyrene (Tsuda and Farber, 1980; Peraino *et al.,* 1981), AAF (Cameron *et al.,* 1978; Pugh and Goldfarb, 1978; Hirota and Williams, 1979; Bibiani and Malvaldi, 1980; Tatematsu *et al.,* 1980; Kuhlmann *et al.,* 1981; Gouy *et al.,* 1983; Capouya and Lindahl, 1983; Sirica *et al.,* 1984), thioacetamide, dimethylaminoazobenzene (DAB) (Taniguchi, 1974; Daoust, 1982), 3′-methyl-DAB (Tateishi *et al.,* 1976; Gotoh *et al.,* 1982), metapyrilene (Oshima *et al.,* 1984), nitrosomorpholine (Boelsterli and Zbinden, 1979; Schulte-Hermann *et al.,* 1981; Moore *et al.,* 1983b; Schwarz *et al.,* 1983), ethionine (Fiala and Fiala, 1973; Schultz-Ellinson *et al.,* 1981), safrole (Lipsky *et al.,* 1980, 1981), *N*-formyl- and *N*-acetyl *N*-hydroxy-4-aminobiphenyl (Shirai *et al.,* 1981), *o*-aminoazotoluene (Jalanko and Ruoslahti, 1979; Kojima *et al.,* 1981), and others.
2. With or without various drugs acting or suspected to act as pro-

moters: DDT (Gouy *et al.*, 1983), Aroclor (Pereira *et al.*, 1982b; Gouy *et al.*, 1983), natural or synthetic hormonal steroids—cortisone, testosterone, cyproterone, norethindrone, mestranol, estradiol, ethinyl estradiol, and morethinodrel (Yager and Yager, 1980; Schuppler *et al.*, 1981; Cameron *et al.*, 1982; Kamden *et al.*, 1983; Yager, 1983), quinoline and ethionine (Tatematsu *et al.*, 1977), bile acids (Cameron *et al.*, 1982), barbital, phenobarbital, barbituric acid, amobarbital (Shinozuka *et al.*, 1982b; Pereira *et al.*, 1982a; Herren and Pereira, 1983), 1,2-dibromoethane (Milks *et al.*, 1982), hexachlorobenzene and lindane (Pereira *et al.*, 1983), hexachlorocyclohexane, metapyrilene (Couri *et al.*, 1982), 3-aminobenzamide (Takahashi *et al.*, 1982a), and others.

3. With or without modifications of the diet: choline-devoid regimen (Sells *et al.*, 1979; Shinozuka *et al.*, 1979, 1982a; Takahashi *et al.*, 1979)

4. Grafted hepatoma cell lines: Morris 5123D, 5123D/AS, and 7777 (Albert, 1979; Fujiwara *et al.*, 1982), Reuber 44 and H139 (Fiala and Reuber, 1970), Novikoff (Wirth and Thorgeirsson, 1978; Fujiwara *et al.*, 1982; Hanigan and Pitot, 1982), Yoshida ascites hepatomas (Tsuchida *et al.*, 1979), RL 34 (Karasaki *et al.*, 1980), HTC, RH 35, ND-HCI, MHC, ARL 16, and ARL 17 (San *et al.*, 1979), HTC, McA-RH7777, and McA-RH8994 (Richards *et al.*, 1982b), and in grafted chemically induced hepatomas (Laishes and Farber, 1978).

1. Kinetics of GGT in Chemically Induced Hepatomas

With most carcinogens, GGT could be evidenced in 10–90% of very early preneoplastic hepatocytes of rat liver. Azoic dyes determined the earliest changes while ethionine had more delayed effects (Huberman *et al.*, 1979; Laishes *et al.*, 1978). With azoic dyes GGT increase could be evidenced before histological disturbances (Bertrand, 1974; Fiala and Fiala, 1971). GGT increased exponentially with time and could reach 10–120 times its normal activity (Fiala *et al.*, 1976).

With DENA, DMBA, and DMH induction and PB promotion, no difference in the number of GGT-positive foci could be attributed to the strain (Fischer 344, Sprague–Dawley, or Wistar Lewis), to the sex, or to the route of administration (oral or intraperitoneal); with DENA, lindane, and hexachlorobenzene, the incidence of GGT-positive foci was higher in female rats (Deml *et al.*, 1981; Pereira *et al.*, 1982b). Meanwhile, partial hepatectomy before DENA stimulation greatly increased the number of GGT-positive foci while it had only minor enhancing effects when performed after DENA stimulation (Hirota *et al.*, 1982; Pereira *et al.*, 1983).

The acute toxicity of AFB_1 and 3′-methyl-DAB was probably responsible for the early diffuse increases of GGT in the periportal zone, and prolonged feeding for 4–6 weeks determined a gradual increase of GGT in clusters of fetal hepatocytes (Fiala *et al.*, 1981; Manson, 1983). Such a liver acute toxicity was also observed with DENA and was considered to play a role in the initial steps of liver carcinogenesis (Ying *et al.*, 1981).

The promoting effect of PB was also observed in spontaneous liver tumors of aged C3HfB/HeN and C3H/HeMsNRS rats in which the discontinuation of PB feeding determined a decrease of GGT (Kitagawa *et al.*, 1980b; Williams *et al.*, 1980).

2. *GGT in Grafted and "Spontaneous" Hepatomas*

In the rat, all hepatomas contained usually at least as much GGT as fetal liver; GGT concentration was not correlated to the rate of tumor growth nor to the differentiation of the cells (Fiala *et al.*, 1976). Few rat hepatomas showed a low GGT concentration, for example, Reuber 44 or Morris 5123D/AS, a fast-growing tumor derived from Morris 5123D line, which contains about 10 times as much GGT (Albert *et al.*, 1977). In aged Fischer 344/NCr rats, PB increased the incidence of GGT-positive foci (Ward, 1983).

In "spontaneous" tumors of mice high GGT was found in only one of four tumors (Fiala *et al.*, 1977; Ohmori *et al.*, 1981). In hamster Kierkman–Robbins hepatoma, GGT concentration was about half that in normal liver (Szewczuk and Albert, 1973).

3. *GGT in Primary Cultures of Adult Rat Hepatocytes*

In 24-hr primary cultures of adult rat hepatocytes, GGT was shown to remain negative (Laishes *et al.*, 1978; Michalopoulos *et al.*, 1982; Lafarge-Frayssinet *et al.*, 1984). When such cultures were maintained for longer periods of time, GGT activity increased steadily with the reversion of the fetal phenotype; GGT was also subject to regulation by various noncarcinogens, thus GGT must be used with caution for *in vitro* hepatocarcinogenesis testing (Sirica *et al.*, 1979; Edwards, 1982; Edwards and Lucas, 1982). In cultures, GGT was increased by moderate doses (1 μmol/liter) of 3′-methyl-DAB, 6-aminochrysene, 3-methylcholanthrene (3-MC), and 2-AAF as well as by 2-methyl-DAB and 2-aminochrysene, which have no *in vivo* cancerogenic activity; on the contrary, GGT was lowered by higher dose (10 and 100 μmol/liter), possibly due to cytotoxicity. The elevation of GGT at low doses was due to generalized increases in every cell (Lowing *et al.*, 1979). Maximum increase was observed about 30–50 hr following a 5 to 10-hr incubation in a medium containing 3-MC.

Rat liver cell lines were not able to metabolize AFB_1, and treatment with this compound did not change GGT content whereas microsomally induced AFB_1 increased GGT level 5- to 10-fold (Manson and Greene, 1982).

GGT was not increased in cultures of liver cells obtained from rats dosed with DEN or DMN (Laishes *et al.*, 1978), but it was high in JBI cells derived from an AFB_1-induced hepatoma (Manson and Green, 1982).

The correlation between GGT expression and cancerogenesis in hepatocytes was also observed in SV40 virus-transformed cells (Laffarge-Frayssinet *et al.*, 1984).

4. *Structure of Liver Carcinoma GGT*

The kinetic, immunological, and molecular characteristics of hepatoma GGT are very similar to those of fetal GGT (Taniguchi *et al.*, 1975): it is a more sialylated protein (Szewczuk *et al.*, 1978; Taniguchi, 1974). The oligosaccharide patterns of AH-66 hepatoma and normal adult hepatocytes are very different: the number of sugar chains per mole of enzyme is greater in hepatoma GGT, which contains more mannose and less sialic acid and also contains bisect *N*-glucosamine residues in 40% of saccharide chains whereas normal liver GGT contains none (Taniguchi, 1974).

5. *Serum GGT in Liver Tumor-Bearing Animals*

In hepatoma-bearing rats or mice, no variation of serum GGT was observed by some authors (Wu *et al.*, 1965; Bertrand, 1974), while others reported significant increases starting on the tenth day (Harada *et al.*, 1976; Albert *et al.*, 1977) and related to the volume of the tumor (Albert, 1976) or the liver GGT content (Mazué *et al.*, 1983). Electrophoresis showed fetal GGT patterns (Harada *et al.*, 1976), while irregular patterns were also obtained according to the tumor and the species (Szewczuk and Albert, 1973). Serum GGT electrophoretic patterns of 5123D, 5123D/AS, and 7777 hepatoma-bearing rats were only slightly different from those of controls (Szewczuk *et al.*, 1982).

In rat, the graft of 5123D Morris hepatoma cells in a limb determines an increase of serum GGT between the third and the fourth week; serum GGT decreased with the removal of the limb then increased again about 10 days later when hepatic metastases occurred (Albert, 1976).

B. GGT IN EXPERIMENTAL NONLIVER TUMORS

Human nephroblastoma cells grafted to nude mice determined a GGT-rich tumor which was responsible for an elevation of serum GGT; the surgical removal of the tumor was followed by a decrease of serum GGT to normal levels (Wise and Muller, 1976).

In mouse mammary carcinoma D 40, GGT was about four times as high as in normal lactating gland (Dawson *et al.*, 1979). In rat mammary carcinoma GGT could be separated by isoelectric focusing from normal tissue enzyme, owing to its higher content in sialic acid (Jaken and Mason, 1978). In rat R 3230 AC mammary tumor, GGT was increased by estradiol but was not as high as in the lactating gland (Suojanen *et al.*, 1980).

The graft of human lung cancer in nude mice induced GGT-rich tumors whereas no GGT could be evidenced in surrounding healthy lung parenchyma (Groscurth *et al.*, 1977).

In mouse skin papillomas GGT was not consistently observed, whereas most squamous carcinoma contained a high concentration of the enzyme (DeYoung *et al.*, 1978; Klein-Szanto *et al.*, 1983).

High GGT activity was also observed in submaxillary carcinomas of the rat; it was not increased in sarcomas (Herzfeld and Raper, 1976).

In golden hamster buccal pouch epithelia, GGT-rich papillomas and squamous carcinomas were shown to develop following topical applications of DMBA (Bernard and Solt, 1982; Solt, 1981; Solt and Shklar, 1982; Odajima *et al.*, 1984) and *N*-methyl-*N*-benzylnitrosamine (Solt *et al.*, 1985).

In the pancreas of the hamster, cancerogenesis was induced by dihydroxy-*n*-propyl- and dioxo-*n*-propyl-nitrosamine, but GGT was only occasionally visible within the regions of atypical proliferations (Moore *et al.*, 1983b).

In rats, *N*-ethyl-*N*-hydroxyethylnitrosamine induced renal cell neoplasms with a marked decrease of GGT activity, which is consistent with a transformation to fetal cell characteristics such as that in liver tumorigenesis but which determines an opposite change of GGT activity (Ohmori *et al.*, 1982).

GGT activity appeared in thyroid atypical proliferations and nodular lesions induced in rats by diisopropylnitrosamine (Moriyama *et al.*, 1983).

V. Urine GGT in Experimental Kidney Toxicity

The bases for the use of enzymes in kidney toxicity have been covered (Price, 1982) elsewhere; therefore, they will not be covered here.

A. Origin of Urine GGT

GGT was first evidenced in human urine (Szewczuk and Orlowski, 1960); then it was also demonstrated in urine of many mammal species. It is postulated to orginate from the kidney and not from the filtration of serum GGT. Such a hypothesis is consistent with the molecular weight of the enzyme, which is greater than the threshold of kidney filtration; moreover, its urinary concentration is not modified in hepatobiliary disturbances and there is no correlation between serum and urine GGT, which exhibit different electrophoretic patterns (Dalal and Winsten, 1973; Mirabile *et al.*, 1973; Thiele, 1973).

B. Assay of Urinary GGT

GGT is stable in urine at room temperature and at 4°C; it is rapidly inactivated by freezing at −20°C (Braun *et al.*, 1978b) but not at −5°C (Rambabu and Pattabiraman, 1976). GGT activity is about 10 times higher in the sediment of rat urine than in the 3000-*g* supernatant (Braun *et al.*, 1978b). In rat urine, urine dialysis does not improve the measurement of GGT activity, although pretreatment of human urines were sometimes recommended (Kley *et al.*, 1973; Bahre *et al.*, 1974; Keyser *et al.*, 1977; Maruhn, 1979; Beck, 1980). The elimination of GGT in urine as well as its kidney concentration exhibit a circadian rhythm; thus, GGT has to be measured in 24-hr urines (Hoffmann and Hardeland, 1981).

Reference values for urine GGT differ with analytical procedures but daily urine GGT was higher in male rats than in females (Braun *et al.*, 1978b).

C. Uses of Urine GGT as a Test of Kidney Toxicity

In experimental toxicology, urine GGT was first used in sheep dosed with mercuric chloride, which determined a very significant increase of GGT excretion during the first day with very great interindividual variations as the basic level was increased about 40- to 140-fold (Shaw, 1976; Robinson and Trafford, 1977).

Most experiments have been carried out in rats dosed with mercuric chloride (Sener *et al.*, 1978; Tsurumi *et al.*, 1978; Koseki *et al.*, 1980; Emmanuelli *et al.*, 1982; Kluwe, 1982), metallic mercury (Burgin *et al.*, 1979), methoxy-ethyl mercury (Burgat *et al.*, 1980), sodium and stannous fluorides (Kessabi *et al.*, 1980, 1981), cadmium (Bonner *et al.*, 1980), *cis*-platinum (Bénard *et al.*, 1981; Dierrickx, 1981; Leyland-Jones *et al., 1983), aspirin (Tsurumi et al.*, 1978; Owen and Heywood, 1980), flufenamic acid, sodium diclofenac, oxyphenbutazone (Tsurumi *et al.*, 1978), ethionine (Durand *et al.*, 1980), folic acid (Maruhn *et al.*, 1981), biphenyl (Kluwe, 1981, 1982), gentamicin and cephaloridine (Inada *et al.*, 1978), kanamycin, neomycin, paramomycin, streptomycin (Dierrickx, 1981), AFB_1 (Grosman *et al.*, 1983), sodium chromate and ethylene imine (Maruhn *et al.*, 1983).

Urine GGT was also demonstrated to be increased by neomycin but not by penicillin treatment in calves (Cromwell *et al.*, 1981), and by mercuric chloride in the horse (Roberts *et al.*, 1982).

With most compounds, the acute proximal toxicity determined a dose-dependent peak increase of urine GGT during the first day following dosage. Fractionated collection of urine every second hour allowed determination of the onset and the duration of the toxic effect due to fluorides (Fig. 1) and to show that stannous fluoride acted longer than the sodium salt (Kessabi *et al.*, 1981). The escape of enzyme from the kidney determined a significant decrease of kidney GGT content in rats dosed either with mercuric chloride (Braun *et al.*, 1978b; Koseki *et al.*, 1980; McEwen-Nicholls *et al.*, 1981), with fluorides (Kessabi *et al.*, 1981), or with gentamicin (Fillastre *et al.*, 1980). In rats given lead acetate, GGT was shown to be significantly lowered within the kidney whereas urine GGT was not significantly changed (McEwen-Nicholls *et al.*, 1983). On the contrary, GGT was increased in kidney brush borders of rats given cadmium (McEwen-Nicholls *et al.*, 1981).

With some drugs—including folates or glafenine (Braun *et al.*, 1981; Maruhn *et al.*, 1981)—GGT excretion was lowered for day 1 of the first two days following dosage, then increased: as both compounds determine obstructive nephropathies, the formation of casts from necrotized tubular cells and their retention could explain the delay of GGT increase.

After the initial increase, GGT usually decreased back to references within 1 or 2 days. In some very severe kidney damage induced by daily repeated administration of mercuric chloride, GGT was shown to

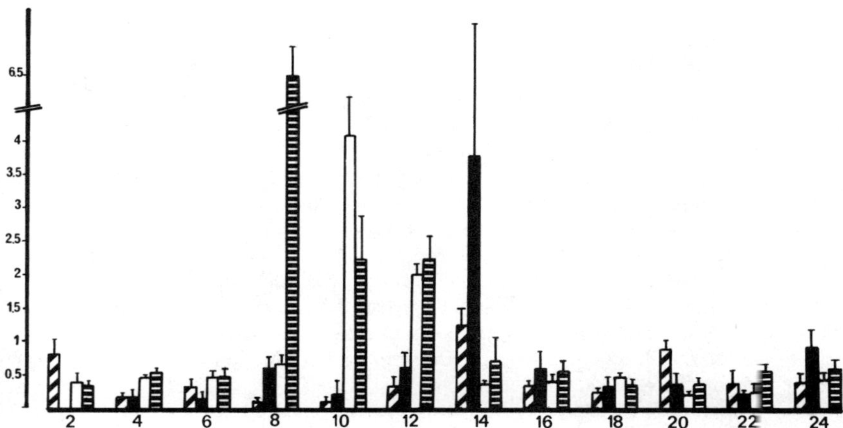

FIG. 1. Dose–effect relationship on 2 hr urine GGT in sheep dosed with sodium fluoride (Kessabi *et al.*, 1981).

be lowered below reference values, probably due to an insufficient regeneration of proximal tubule epithelia (Sener *et al.*, 1979).

VI. Conclusion

In experimental toxicology GGT measurements have become routine tests in the following situations:

1. Hepatic induction testing, whereas toxic liver necrosis only has applications limited to some species such as ruminants and horses;
2. Carcinogenesis in rodents, where it is one of the earliest and most sensitive tests of hepatocellular transformation;
3. Nephrotoxicity testing, in which it is a good marker of proximal tubular damage.

But there are many intra- and interindividual variations. The control of all the factors of variation need more fundamental research. It seems more and more clear that all three types of experimental toxicology uses of GGT involve the intracellular communication role of this sialylated glycoprotein. Furthermore, the hormonal regulation of the enzyme could play a greater role than suspected and, finally, the knowledge of molecular mechanisms of GGT induction, as compared to those of drug-metabolizing enzymes, should provide a better basis for the interpretation of the enzyme.

References

Adjarov, D., Ivanov, E., and Keremidchiev, D. (1982). *Toxicology* **23,** 73.
Albert, M. (1979). *Folia Histochem. Cytochem.* **17,** 363.
Albert, W. (1976). *Folia Histochem. Cytochem.* **14,** 181.
Albert, Z., Orlowska, J., Orlowski, M., and Szewczuk, A. (1964). *Acta Histochem.* **18,** 78.
Albert, Z., Szewczuk, A., and Albert, W. (1977). *Neoplasma* **24,** 49.
Appleton, B. S., and Campbell, T. C. (1983). *Cancer Res.* **43,** 2150.
Artur, Y., Wellmann-Benawska, M., and Siest, G. (1984). *Ann. Biol. Clin.* **42,** 115.
Badylak, S. F., and Van Vleet, J. F. (1982). *Am. J. Vet. Res.* **43,** 649.
Bagrel, D., Ratanasavahn, D., and Siest, G. (1980). *Pharmacol. Res. Commun.* **12,** 557.
Bahre, G., Kley, R., and Brass, H. (1974). *Dtsch. Med. Wochenschr.* **99,** 2114.
Beck, P. (1980). *In* "Progress in Clinical Enzymology" (D. M. Goldberg and M. Werner, eds.). Masson, New York.
Bénard, P., Braun, J. P., Maquet, J. P., Burgat, V., and Rico, A. G. (1981). *In* "Organ Directed Toxicity. Chemical Indices and Mechanisms" (S. Brown and S. S. Davies, eds.). Pergamon, Oxford.
Bernard, D. P., and Solt, D. B. (1982). *In* "Safety Evaluation and Regulation of Chemicals" (F. Homburger, ed.), pp. 173–182. Karger, Basel.
Bertrand, L. (1974). *In* "Apport de la détermination de la Gamma-glutamyl transpeptidase en sémiologie hépatique," pp. 49–52. Boehringer, Paris.
Bézille, P., Braun, J. P., and LeBars, J. (1984). *Rec. Med. Vet.* **160,** 339.
Bibiani, C., and Malvaldi, G. (1980). *Boll. Soc. Ital. Biol. Sper.* **56,** 1722.
Boelsterli, U., and Zbinden, G. (1979). *Arch. Toxicol.* **42,** 225.
Bonner, F. W., King, L. J., and Parke, D. V. (1980). *Environ. Res.* **22,** 237.
Boyd, J. N., Stowsand, G. S., Misslbeck, N., Campbell, T. C., Mason, R., Lepp, C. A., and Odstrechl, G. (1981). *J. Toxicol. Environ. Health* **7,** 1025.
Braun, J. P., and Fernet, P. (1982). *Pathol. Biol.* **30,** 243.
Braun, J. P., Rico, A. G., Bénard, P., and Burgat-Sacaze, V. (1977). *Ann. Biol. Clin.* **35,** 433.
Braun, J. P., Rico, A. G., and Bénard, P. (1978a). *C.R. Acad. Sci. Paris* **286D,** 1483.
Braun, J. P., Rico, A. G., Bénard, P., Burgat-Sacaze, V., Eghbali, B., and Godfrain, J. C. (1978b). *Toxicology* **11,** 73.
Braun, J. P., Burgat, V., Bénard, P., and Rico, A. G. (1982). *In* "Gamma-glutamyl Transférases" (G. Siest, and C. Heusghem, eds.), pp. 185–193. Masson, Paris.
Braun, J. P., Rico, A. G., Bénard, P., and Burgat, V. (1980). *J. Med. Primatol.* **9,** 185.
Braun, J. P., Delmon, A., Bénard, P., Burgat, V., and Rico, A. (1981). *Gen. Pharmacol.* **12,** A35.
Burgat, V., Braun, J. P., Rico, A. G., Bénard, P., and Eghbali, B. (1980). *Arch. Toxicol.* **43,** 227.
Burgin, H., Knutti, R., Zbinden, G., and Schlatter, C. (1979). *Congr. Eur. Soc. Toxicol., 21st, Dresden.*
Cameron, R., Kellen, J., Kolin, A., Malkin, A., and Farber, E. (1978). *Cancer Res.* **38,** 823.
Cameron, R. G., Imaida, K., Tsuda, H., and Ito, N. (1982). *Cancer Res.* **42,** 2426.
Capouya, E. R., and Lindahl, R. (1983). *J. Natl. Cancer Inst.* **70,** 359.
Collis, K. A., and Stark, A. J. (1977). *Res. Vet. Sci.* **23,** 326.
Colombo, J. P., and Gigon, P. L. (1979). *Experientia* **35,** 1005.
Colona, J., Gomez-Lechon, M. J., Garcia, M. D., Feliu, E., and Baguena, J. (1981). *Experientia* **37,** 941.

Columbano, A., Ledda, G. M., Rao, P. M., Rajalakshmi, S., and Sarma, D. S. R. (1982). *Cancer Lett.* **16,** 191.
Couri, D., Wilt, S. R., and Milks, M. M. (1982). *Res. Commun. Chem. Pathol. Pharmacol.* **35,** 51.
Cromwell, W. A., Divers, T. J., Byars, T. D., Marshall, A. E., Nusbaum, K. E., and Larsen, L. (1981). *Am. J. Vet. Res.* **42,** 29.
Dalal, F. B., and Winsten, S. (1973). *Clin. Chem.* **78,** 499.
Daoust, R. (1982). *J. Histochem. Cytochem.* **4,** 312.
Dawson, J., Smith, G. D., Boak, J., and Petres, T. J. (1979). *Clin. Chim. Acta* **96,** 37.
Deml, E., Oesterle, D., Wolff, T., and Greim, H. (1981). *J. Cancer Res. Clin. Oncol.* **100,** 125.
DeNovo, R. C., and Prasse, K. W. (1983). *Am. J. Vet. Res.* **44,** 1703.
DeYoung, L. M., Richards, W. L., Bonzelet, W., Tsai, L. L., and Boutwell, T. (1978). *Cancer Res.* **38,** 3697.
Dierickx, P. J. (1981). *Arch. Toxicol.* **47,** 209.
Durand, S., Bénard, P., and Braun, J. P. (1980). *Toxicol. Lett.* **5,** 257.
Edwards, A. M. (1982). *Cancer Res.* **42,** 1107.
Edwards, A. M., and Lucas, C. M. (1982). *In* "*In vitro* Epithelial Cell Differentiation and Neoplasia" (G. J. Smith and B. W. Stewart, eds.), pp. 173–191. Australian Cancer Society, Sidney.
Emmanuelli, G., Cestonaro, G., Anfossi, G., Calcamuggi, G., Gatti, G., and Marcarino, C. (1982). *Enzyme* **27,** 89.
Faeder, E. J., Chaney, S. Q., King, L. C., Hinners, T. A., Bruce, R., and Fowler, B. A. (1977). *Toxicol. Appl. Pharmacol.* **39,** 473.
Fiala, S., and Fiala, A. E. (1969). *Naturwissenschaften* **56,** 565.
Fiala, S., Fiala, A. E., and Dixon, R. (1972). *J. Natl. Cancer Inst.* **48,** 1393.
Fiala, S., and Fiala, E. S. (1971). *Naturwissenschaften* **58,** 330.
Fiala, S., and Fiala, E. S. (1973). *J. Natl. Cancer Inst.* **51,** 151.
Fiala, S., and Reuber, M. D. (1970). *Gann* **61,** 275.
Fiala, S., Mohindru, A., Kettering, W. G., Fiala, A. E., and Morris, H. P. (1976). *J. Natl. Cancer Inst.* **57,** 591.
Fiala, S., Fiala, A. E., Keller, R. W., and Fiala, E. S. (1977). *Arch. Geschwülstforsch.* **47,** 117.
Fiala, S., Pragani, B., and Reuber, M. D. (1978). *Tumori* **64,** 131.
Fiala, S., Fiala, A., Kettering, W., and Trout, E. (1981). *Cancer Res.* **22,** 73.
Fillastre, J. P., Godin, M., Morin, J. P., Bendirdjian, J. P., and Viotte, G. (1980). *In* "La fonction rénale" (J. P. Bonvalet, ed.), pp. 223–249. INSERN Flammarion Paris.
Findeisen, R. (1972). Inaug. dissertation Vet. Med., Hannover.
Floersheim, G. L., Eberhard, M., Tschumi, P., and Duckert, F. (1978). *Toxicol. Appl. Pharmacol.* **46,** 455.
Ford, E. J. H. (1974). *J. Comp. Pathol.* **84,** 231.
Ford, E. J. H., and Adam, P. (1981). *Res. Vet. Sci.* **31,** 312.
Ford, J. O., and Pereira, M. A. (1980). *J. Environ. Pathol. Toxicol.* **4,** 39.
Fujiwara, K., Katyal, S. L., and Lombardi, B. (1982). *Enzyme* **27,** 114.
Galteau, M. M., Siest, G., and Ratanasavahn, D. (1980). *Cell. Mol. Biol.* **26,** 267.
Garcia, M. B., and Mourelle, M. (1984). *J. Appl. Toxicol.* **4,** 246.
Garthoff, L. H., Cerra, F. E., and Marks, E. M. (1981). *Toxicol. Appl. Pharmacol.* **60,** 33.
Gibinski, K., and Aleksandrowitch, J. (1965). *Arch. Immunol. Ther. Exp.* **13,** 557.
Goldberg, D. M. (1980). *CRC Crit. Rev. Clin. Lab. Sci.* **12,** 1.
Goldberg, D. M., Yu, A., Roomi, M. W., and Roncari, D. A. K. (1981). *Can. J. Biochem.* **59,** 48.

Gotoh, M., Mochizuki, Y., Furukawa, K., Sawada, N., and Tsukada, H. (1982). *Gann* **73,** 14.
Gouy, D., Remandet, B., Garbay, J. M., Berthe, J., and Mazué, G. (1983). *Biol. Prospect. Colloq. Int., 5th, Pont-à-Mousson.*
Groscurth, P., Fleming, N., and Kistler, G. S. (1977). *Proc. Natl. Acad. Sci. U.S.A.* **53,** 135.
Grosman, M. E., Elias, M. M., Comin, E. J., and Garay, E. A. R. (1983). *Toxicol. Appl. Pharmacol.* **69,** 319.
Hanigan, H. M., and Pitot, H. C. (1982). *Carcinogenesis* **11,** 1349.
Harada, M., Okabe, K., Shibata, K., Masuda, H., Miyata, K., and Enomodo, M. (1976). *Acta Histochem. Cytochem.* **9,** 168.
Heinle, H., Wendel, A., and Schmidt, U. (1977). *Arch. Immunol. Ther. Exp.* **18,** 185.
Herren, S. L., and Pereira, M. A. (1983). *Environ. Health Perspect.* **50,** 123.
Herzfeld, A., and Raper, S. M. (1976). *Enzyme* **21,** 471.
Hirota, N., and Williams, G. M. (1979). *Am. J. Pathol.* **95,** 317.
Hirota, N., Moriyama, S., and Yokoyama, T. (1982). *J. Natl. Cancer Inst.* **69,** 1299.
Hoffmann, J., and Hardeland, R. (1981). *Arch. Int. Physiol. Biochem.* **89,** 245.
Huberman, E., Montesano, R., Drevon, C., Kuroki, T., Saint-Vincent, L., Pugh, T. D., and Goldfaris, S. (1979). *J. Natl. Cancer Inst.* **39,** 269.
Huseby, N. E. (1979). *Clin. Chim. Acta* **94,** 163.
Ideo, G., DeFranchis, R., DelNino, E., and Dioguardi, N. (1971). *Lancet,* **II,** 825.
Ideo, G., Morganti, A., and Dioguardi, N. (1972). *Digestion* **5,** 326.
Igarashi, S., Satoh, T., Ueno, K., and Kitagawa, H. (1981). *Life Sci.* **29,** 483.
Igarashi, T., Satoh, T., Hoshi, K., Ueno, K., and Kitagawa, H. (1982). *Life Sci.* **31,** 2655.
Ikeda, S., Yamaoka, S., Watanabe, H., and Kameya, T. (1976). *Exp. Rep. Equine Health Lab.* **13,** 1.
Inada, Y., Terashita, Z., Shibouta, Y., Ando, T., Shimakawa, H., Nishikawa, K., Kikuchi, S., and Shimamoto, K. (1978). *J. Takeda Res. Lab.* **37,** 41.
Ivanov, E., Krustev, L., Adjarov, D., Chernev, K., Apostolow, I., Dimitrov, P., Drenska, E., Stefanova, M., and Pramatarova, V. (1976). *Enzyme* **21,** 8.
Jaken, S., and Mason, M. (1978). *Proc. Natl. Acad. Sci. U.S.A.* **75,** 1750.
Jalanko, H., and Ruoslahti, E. (1979). *Cancer Res.* **39,** 3495.
Jedrzejewski, K., and Kugler, P. (1982). *Histochemistry* **74,** 63.
Kamden, L., Magdalou, J., and Siest, G. (1981). *Toxicol. Appl. Pharmacol.* **60,** 570.
Kamden, L., Magdalou, J., and Siest, G. (1982). *In* "Gamma-glutamyl Transférases" (G. Siest and C. Heusghem, eds.), pp. 115–120. Masson, Paris.
Kamden, L., Magdalou, J., Siest, G., Ban, M., and Zissu, D. (1983). *Toxicol. Appl. Pharmacol.* **67,** 26.
Karasaki, S., Suh, M. H., Salas, M., and Raymond, J. (1980). *Cancer Res.* **40,** 1318.
Keller, P. (1981). *Am. J. Vet. Res.* **42,** 575.
Kessabi, M., Braun, J. P., Bénard, P., Burgat, V., and Rico, A. G. (1980). *Toxicol. Lett.* **5,** 169.
Kessabi, M., Braun, J. P., Burgat, V., Bénard, P., and Rico, A. G. (1981). *Toxicol. Lett.* **7,** 463.
Keyser, J. W., Watkins, G. L., and Salaman, J. R. (1977). *Clin. Chem.* **13,** 770.
Kitagawa, T., Inai, F., and Sato, K. (1980a). *Gann* **71,** 362.
Kitagawa, T., Watanabe, R., and Sugano, H. (1980b). *Gann* **71,** 536.
Klein-Szanto, A. J. P., Nelso, K. G., Shah, Y., and Slaga, T. J. (1983). *J. Natl. Cancer Inst.* **70,** 161.
Kley, R., Bahre, G., and Holzhuter, H. (1973). *Z. Klin. Chem. Klin. Biochem.* **11,** 537.
Kluwe, W. M. (1981). *Toxicol. Appl. Pharmacol.* **57,** 414.

Kluwe, W. M. (1982). *J. Toxicol. Environ. Health* **9,** 619.
Kojima, S., Hama, Y., and Kubodera, A. (1981). *Toxicol. Appl. Pharmacol.* **60,** 26.
Koseki, C., Endou, H., Sudo, J. I., Shimada, H., and Sakai, F. (1980). *Folia Pharmacol. Jpn.* **76,** 59.
Kuhlmann, W. D., Krischan, R., Kunz, W., Guenthner, T. M., and Oesch, F. (1981). *Biochem. Biophys. Res. Commun.* **98,** 417.
Kuska, J., and Kokot, F. (1970). *Arch. Immunol. Ther. Exp.* **18,** 185.
Lafarge-Frayssinet, C., Estrade, S., Rosa-Loridon, B., Frayssinet, C., and Cassigena, R. (1984). *Cancer Lett.* **22,** 31.
Laishes, B. A., and Farber, E. (1978). *J. Natl. Cancer Inst.* **61,** 507.
Laishes, B. A., Ogawa, K., Roberts, E., and Farber, E. (1978). *J. Natl. Cancer Inst.* **60,** 1009.
Lamy, J., Baglin, M. C., Weill, J., and Aron, E. (1975). *Nouv. Presse Méd.* **4,** 487.
Lavinski, M. (1968). *Arch. Immunol. Ther. Exp.* **16,** 942.
Levanti, G., Fehlmann, M., Starita-Geribaldi, M., and Sudaka, P. (1978). *Arch. Biol. Anim. Biochim. Biophys.* **18,** 1155.
Leyland-Jones, B., Morrow, C., Tate, S., Urmacher, C., Gordon, C., and Young, C. W. (1983). *Cancer Res.* **43,** 6072.
Lipsky, M. M., Hinton, D. E., Klaunig, J. E., Goldblatt, P. J., and Trump, B. F. (1980). *Carcinogenesis* **1,** 151.
Lipsky, M. M., Hinton, D. E., Klaunig, J. E., Goldblatt, P. J., and Trump, B. F. (1981). *J. Natl. Cancer Inst.* **67,** 377.
Lowing, R. Y., Fry, J. R., Jones, C. A., Wiebkin, P., King, L. J., and Bridges, J. W. (1979). *Chem. Biol. Interact.* **24,** 121.
McEwen-Nicholls, D., Teichert-Kuliszewska, K., and Kuliszewski, M. J. (1981). *Toxicol. Appl. Pharmacol.* **61,** 441.
McEwen-Nicholls, D., Teichert-Kuliszewska, K., and Kuliszewski, M. J. (1983). *Toxicol. Appl. Pharmacol.* **67,** 193.
Majumder, G. C., and Ganguli, N. C. (1972). *Milchwissenschaft* **27,** 484.
Malherbe, W. D., Kellerman, T. S., Kriek, N. P. J., and Haupt, W. H. (1977). *Onderstepoort J. Vet. Res.* **44,** 29.
Malyusz, M., and Ehrens, H. J. (1983). *Enzyme* **19,** 93.
Manson, M. M. (1983). *Carcinogenesis* **4,** 467.
Manson, M. M., and Green, J. A. (1982). *Br. J. Cancer* **45,** 945.
Maruhn, D. (1979). *In* "Diagnostic Significance of Proteins and Enzymes in Urine" (L. C. Dubach and U. Schmidt, eds.), pp. 22–30. Hüber, Bern.
Maruhn, D., Paar, D., Hartmann, M. G., Bock, K. D., Bomhard, E., and Lorke, D. (1981). *In* "Organ-directed Toxicity. Chemical Indices and Mechanisms" (S. S. Brown and D. C. Davies, eds.), pp. 697–73. Pergamon, Oxford.
Maruhn, D., Paar, D., and Bomhard, E. (1983). *Biol. Prospect., Colloq. Int., 5th, Pont-à-Mousson.*
Mazué, G., Gouy, D., and Remandet, B. (1983). *In* "Safety Evaluation and Regulation of Chemicals" (F. Homburger, ed.), pp. 251–258. Karger, Basel.
Meyer, D. J. (1982). *J. Am. Anim. Hosp. Assoc.* **18,** 725.
Meyer, D. J., and Noonan, N. E. (1981). *J. Am. Anim. Hosp. Assoc.* **17,** 261.
Michalopoulos, G., Cianciulli, H. D., Novotny, A. R., Kligerman, A. D., Strom, S. C., and Jirtle, R. L. (1982). *Cancer Res.* **42,** 4673.
Milks, M. M., Wilt, S. R., Ali, I., Pereira, M. A., and Couri, D. (1982). *Arch. Toxicol.* **51,** 27.
Mirabile, V., Bitto, T., Uziel, L., Tornaghi, G., and Ideo, G. (1973). *Quad. Sclavo Diagn. Clin. Lab.* **9,** 374.

Moore, M. A., Hacker, H. J., Kunz, H. W., and Bannasch, P. (1983a). *Carcinogenesis* **4,** 473.
Moore, M. A., Takahashi, M., Ito, N., and Bannasch, P. (1983b). *Carcinogenesis* **4,** 431.
Moriyama, S., Kawaoi, A., and Hirota, N. (1983). *Brit. J. Cancer* **47,** 299.
Müller, E., Colombo, J. P., Peheim, E., and Bircher, J. (1974). *Experientia* **30,** 1128.
Naftalin, L., Child, V. J., Morlay, D. A., and Smith, D. A. (1969). *Clin. Chim. Acta* **26,** 297.
Noonan, N. E. (1981). *Am. J. Vet. Res.* **42,** 674.
Odajima, T., Solt, D. B., and Solt, L. C. (1984). *Cancer Res.* **44,** 2062.
Ogawa, K., Onoe, T., and Takuchi, M. (1981). *J. Natl. Cancer Inst.* **67,** 407.
Ohmori, T., Rice, J. M., and Williams, G. M. (1981). *Histochem. J.* **13,** 85.
Ohmori, T., Hiasa, Y., Murata, Y., and Williams, G. M. (1982). *Gann* **73,** 543.
Ohshima, M., Ward, J. M., Brenan, L. M., and Creasia, D. A. (1984). *J. Natl. Cancer Inst.* **72,** 759.
Onoé, T., Kaneko, A., Yoshida, Y., Dempo, K., Chisaka, N., Yokoyama, S., and Ogawa, K. (1976). *In* "Onco-developmental Gene Expression" (W. H. Fishmann and S. Sell, eds.). Academic Press, New York.
Owen, R. A., and Heywood, R. (1980). *Toxicol. Lett.* **5,** 269.
Palyza, V., Pinka, J., Kulhanek, V., and Janosek, S. (1969). *Z. Inn. Med.* **24,** 273.
Peraino, C., Staffeldt, E. F., and Ludeman, V. N. (1981). *Carcinogenesis* **2,** 463.
Pereira, M. A., Herren, S. L., Britt, A. L., and Khoury, M. M. (1982a). *Cancer Lett.* **15,** 95.
Pereira, M. A., Herren, S. L., Britt, A. L., and Khoury, M. M. (1982b). *Cancer Lett.* **15,** 185.
Pereira, M. A., Savage, R. E., Herren, S. L., and Guion, C. W. (1982c). *Carcinogenesis* **3,** 147.
Pereira, M. A., Herren-Freund, S. L., Britt, A. L., and Khoury, M. M. (1983). *Cancer Lett.* **20,** 207.
Pereira, M. A., Herren-Freund, S. L., Britt, A. L., and Khoury, M. M. (1984). *J. Natl. Cancer Inst.* **72,** 741.
Pitot, H. C., Barsness, L., Goldsworthy, T., and Kitagawa, T. (1978). *Nature (London)* **271,** 456.
Price, R. G. (1982). *Toxicology* **23,** 99.
Pugh, T. D., and Goldfarb, S. (1978). *Cancer Res.* **38,** 4450.
Rambabu, K., and Pattabiraman, T. N. (1976). *Clin. Chim. Acta* **73,** 251.
Ratanasavahn, D., Magdalou, J., Antoine, B., Galteau, M. M., and Siest, G. (1981). *Pharmacol. Res. Commun.* **13,** 909.
Ratanasavahn, D., Tazi, A., Gaspart, E., Jaquier, A., Notter, D., Galteau, M. M., and Siest, G. (1982). *In* "Gamma-glutamyl Transferases" (G. Siest and C. Heusghem, eds.), pp. 93–103. Masson, Paris.
Ratanasavahn, D., Houssier, M., Galteau, M. M., and Siest, G. (1984). *Clin. Chim. Acta* **144,** 127.
Richards, W. L., Tsukada, Y., and van Potter, R. (1982a). *Cancer Res.* **43,** 1374.
Richards, W. L., Tsukada, Y., and van Potter, R. (1982b). *Cancer Res.* **42,** 5133.
Rico, A. G., Braun, J. P., Bénard, P., and Thouvenot, J. P. (1977). *J. Dairy Sci.* **60,** 1283.
Roberts, M. C., Seawright, A. A., and Norman, P. D. (1982). *Vet. Hum. Toxicol.* **24,** 415.
Robinson, M., and Trafford, J. (1977). *J. Comp. Med.* **87,** 275.
Roomi, M. W., and Goldberg, D. M. (1981). *Biochem. Pharmacol.* **30,** 1563.
Rosalki, S. B. (1974). *Am. J. Clin. Pathol.* **62,** 579.
Rosalki, S. B. (1975). *Adv. Clin. Chem.* **17,** 53.
Rosalki, S. B. (1977). *Rev. Epidemiol. Santé Publ.* **25,** 147.
Rosenberg, M. R., Strom, S. C., and Michalopoulos, G. (1982). *In Vitro* **18,** 775.
Roushdy, H. M., and Mansour, M. A. (1980). *Ann. Zool.* **16,** 89.

Rumler, W., Grundig, C. A., and Maaz, H. J. (1972). *Acta Biol. Med. Germ* **29,** 259.
San, R. H. C., Shimada, T., Maslansky, C. J., Kreiser, D. M., Laspia, M. F., Rice, J. M., and Williams, G. M. (1979). *Cancer Res.* **39,** 4441.
Sassowa, J. (1968). *Arch. Immunol. Ther. Exp.* **16,** 659.
Satoh, T., Igarashi, T., Hirota, T., and Kitagawa, H. (1982). *J. Pharmacol. Exp. Ther.* **221** 795.
Sawada, N., Furukawa, K., and Tsukuda, H. (1982). *J. Natl. Cancer Inst.* **69,** 683.
Scherberich, J. E., and Gauhl, C. U. M. (1978). *In* "Biochemical Nephrology" (W. G. Guder and U. Schmidt, eds.), pp. 426–436. Hüber, Bern.
Scherberich, J. E., Stefanescu, T., Mondorf, W., and Falkenberg, F. (1978). *In* "Chromatography of Synthetic and Natural Material" (R. Epton, ed.), pp. 314–324. Ellis Horwood, Chichester.
Schmidt, E., and Schmidt, F. W. (1973). *Dtsch. Med. Wochenschr.* **98,** 1572.
Schulte-Hermann, R., Ohde, G., Schuppler, J., and Timmermann-Trosenier, I. (1981). *Cancer Res.* **41,** 2556.
Schultz-Ellison, G., Atryzek, V., and Fausto, N. (1981). *Oncodev. Biol. Med.* **2,** 109.
Schuppler, J., Damme, J., and Schulte-Hermann, R. (1981). *Carcinogenesis* **2,** 239.
Schwarz, M., Bannasch, P., and Kuntz, W. (1983). *Cancer Lett.* **21,** 17.
Sekas, G., and Cook, R. T. (1979). *Br. J. Exp. Pathol.* **60,** 447.
Sells, M. A., Katyal, S. L., Sell, S., Shinozuka, H., and Lombardi, B. (1979). *Br J. Cancer* **40,** 274.
Sener, S., Braun, J. P., Rico, A. G., Bénard, P., and Burgat, V. (1978). *Toxicol. Eur. Res.* **4,** 263.
Sener, S., Braun, J. P., Rico, A. G., Bénard, P., and Burgat, V. (1979). *Toxicology* **12,** 299.
Shaw, F. D. (1976). *Res. Vet. Sci.* **20,** 226.
Shimada, H., Endou, H., and Sakai, F. (1982). *Jpn. J. Pharmacol.* **32,** 121.
Shinozuka, H., Sells, M. A., Katyal, S. L., Sell, S., and Lombardi, B. (1979). *Cancer Res.* **39,** 2515.
Shinozuka, H., Lombardi, B., and Abanobi, S. E. (1982a). *Carcinogenesis* **3,** 1017.
Shinozuka, H., Takahashi, S., Lombardi, B., and Abanobi, S. E. (1982b). *Cancer Lett.* **16,** 43.
Shirai, T., Lee, M. S., Wang, C. W., and King, C. M. (1981). *Cancer Res.* **41,** 2450.
Siest, G., and Heusghem, C., eds. (1982). "Gamma-glutamyl Transferases." Masson, Paris.
Siest, G., Bagrel, D., Ratanasavahn, D., Galteau, M. M., Tazi, A., Schiele, F., and Petitclerc, C. (1980). *In* "Industrial and Clinical Enzymology" (L. Vitale and V. Simeon, eds.), pp. 193–201. Pergamon, Oxford.
Siest, G., Ratanasavahn, D., Galteau, M. M., Houssier, M., Antoine, B., and Batt, A. M. (1982a). *In* "Advances in Biochemical Pharmacology, 3rd series" (G. Siest and C. Heusghem, eds.), pp. 73–79. Masson, Paris.
Siest, G., Ratanasavahn, D., Galteau, M. M., and Wellmann-Bednavska, M. (1982b). *In* "Cell Function and Differentiation (G. Akoyonoglon, A. E. Evangelopoulos, J. Georgotos, G. Palaiologos, A. Tcakatellis, C. P. Tsiganos, eds.), pp. 409–421. Liss, New York.
Sirica, A. E., Richards, W., Tsukuda, Y., Sattler, C. A., and Pitot, H. C. (1979). *Proc. Natl. Acad. Sci. U.S.A.* **76,** 283.
Sirica, A. E., Jicinsky, J. K., and Heyer, E. K. (1984). *Carcinogenesis* **5,** 1737.
Sledzinski, Z., and Kokot, F. (1977). *Arch. Immunol. Ther. Exp.* **25,** 601.
Sobiech, K. A., and Szewczuk, A. (1974). *Arch. Immunol. Ther. Exp.* **22,** 635.
Solt, D. B. (1981). *J. Natl. Cancer Inst.* **67,** 193.
Solt, D. B., and Shklar, G. (1982). *Cancer Res.* **42,** 285.
Solt, D. B., Calderon-Solt, L., and Odajima. T. (1985). *J. Natl. Cancer Inst.* **74,** 437.

Stout, D. L., and Becker, F. F. (1982). *Carcinogenesis* **3,** 599.
Suojanen, J. N., Gay, R. J., and Hilf, R. (1980). *Biochem. Biophys. Acta* **630,** 485.
Szacki, J., and Lavinski, M. (1969). *Arch. Immunol. Ther. Exp.* **17,** 823.
Szasz, G. (1974). *In* "Methods of Enzymatic Analysis" (H. U. Bergmeyer, ed.), pp. 715–723. Academic Press, New York.
Szewczuk, A., and Albert, Z. (1973). *Folia Histochem. Cytochem.* **11,** 75.
Szewczuk, A., and Orlowski, M. (1960). *Clin. Chim. Acta* **5,** 680.
Szewczuk, A., Milnerowicz, H., and Sobiech, K. A. (1978). *Neoplasma* **25,** 297.
Szewczuk, A., Milnerowicz, H., Prusak, E., and Albert, Z. (1982). *Folia Histochem. Cytochem.* **20,** 25.
Takahashi, S., Katyal, S. L., Lombardi, B., and Shinozuka, H. (1979). *Cancer Lett.* **7,** 265.
Takahashi, S., Lombardi, B., and Shinozuka, H. (1982a). *Int. J. Cancer* **29,** 445.
Takahashi, S., Ohnishi, T., Denda, A., and Konishi, Y. (1982b). *Chem. Biol. Interact.* **39,** 363.
Taniguchi, N. (1974). *J. Biochem.* **75,** 473.
Taniguchi, N. (1975). *J. Biochem.* **76,** 381.
Taniguchi, N., Saoto, K., and Takakjwa, E. (1975). *Biochim. Biophys. Acta* **391,** 265.
Tate, S. S., and Meister, A. (1981). *Mol. Cell. Biochem.* **39,** 357.
Tateishi, N., Higashi, T., Nomura, T., Naruse, A., Nakashima, K., Shozaki, H., and Sakamoto, Y. (1976). *Gann* **67,** 215.
Tatematsu, M., Shirai, T., Tsuda, H., Miyata, Y., Shinohara, Y., and Ito, N. (1977). *Gann* **68,** 499.
Tatematsu, M., Takano, T., Hasegawa, R., Imaida, K., Nakanowatari, J., and Ito, N. (1980). *Gann* **71,** 843.
Tazi, A., Galteau, M. M., and Siest, G. (1980). *Toxicol. Appl. Pharmacol.* **55,** 1.
Thiele, K. G. (1973). *Klin. Wochenschr.* **51,** 339.
Towers, N. R., and Smith, B. L. (1978). *N.Z. Vet. J.* **26,** 199.
Towers, N. R., and Stratton, G. S. (1978). *N.Z. Vet. J.* **26,** 109.
Tsao, B., and Curthoys, N. P. (1982). *Biochim. Biophys. Acta* **690,** 199.
Tsuchida, S., Hoshino, K., Sato, T., Ito, N., and Sato, K. (1979). *Cancer Res.* **39,** 4200.
Tsuda, H., and Farber E. (1980). *Int. J. Cancer* **25,** 137.
Tsuda, H., Hasegawa, R., Imaida, K., Masui, T., Moore, M. A., and Ito, N. (1984). *Gann* **75,** 876.
Tsurumi, K., Abe, A., Nozaki, M., and Fujimura, H. (1978). *J. Toxicol. Sci.* **3,** 1.
Wapnir, R. A., Macusi, V. J., and Goldstein, L. A. (1982). *Experientia* **38,** 647.
Ward, J. M. (1983). *Cancer Res.* **71,** 815.
Williams, G. M., Ohmori, T., Katayama, S., and Rice, J. M. (1980). *Carcinogenesis* **1,** 813.
Wirth, P. J., and Thorgeirsson, S. S. (1978). *Cancer Res.* **38,** 2861.
Wise, K. S., and Muller, E. (1976). *Experientia* **32,** 294.
Wu, C., Roberts, E., and Bauer, J. M. (1965). *Cancer Res.* **25,** 677.
Yager, J. D. (1983). *Environ. Health Perspect.* **50,** 109.
Yager, J. D., and Yager, R. (1980). *Cancer Res.* **40,** 3680.
Yager, J. D., Campbell, H. A., Longnecker, D. S., Roebuck, B. D., and Benoit, M. C. (1984). *Cancer Res.* **44,** 3862.
Yamashita, K., Hitoi, A., Taniguchi, N., Yokosawa, N., Tsukuda, Y., and Kobata, A. (1983). *Cancer Res.* **43,** 5059.
Ying, T. S., Sarma, D. S. R., and Farber, E. (1981). *Cancer Res.* **41,** 2096.
Ying, T. S., Enomoto, K., Sarma, D. S. R., and Farber, E. (1982). *Cancer Res.* **42,** 876.
Yonaba, M., Ishikura, S., and Uchiyama, M. (1975). *Chem. Pharmacol. Bull.* **23,** 1726.
Zawirska, B. (1982). *Neoplasma* **29,** 693.

Predictive Value of Ocular Irritation Tests

PIERRE DUPRAT* AND PHILIPPE CONQUET†

*Centre de Recherche, Laboratoires Merck Sharp & Dohme-Chibret, Route de Marsat, 63203 Riom Cedex, France

†Laboratoires Merck Sharp & Dohme-Chibret, 3 Avenue Hoche, 75 008 Paris, France

I. Introduction

A wide variety of drugs, cosmetics, and chemicals are likely to come into contact with the eye and adnexa, either after deliberate administration or by chance or accident. Consequently, the evaluation of their potential for ocular irritation is an essential and legally required step in their development. Historically, the rabbit has been the empirical choice for providing this information, using methodologies relying on clinical evaluation of eye damage, subjectively ranked, and leading to a final score composed of added dissimilar, nonparametric data. For many regulatory agencies, the Draize test (1944) with successive modifications has become the test of choice. However, this procedure is questionable not only from a statistical viewpoint; it also has been shown to lack sensitivity and reproducibility (Weltman *et al.*, 1965). In addition, the amount of each compound administered by requirement, regardless of its physicochemical properties, can provoke dramatic reactions and unnecessary pain leading to meaningless results. That is why this test has been sharply criticized, and many attempts are being made throughout the world to develop alternatives for predictive ocular irritancy as is shown by the rapidly increasing number of publications on this subject.

With regard to ophthalmic preparations the situation is radically different, even if basically the evaluation of their potential for ocular irritation remains subjective and based on clinical evaluation as for the Draize test. This is because these preparations are developed for deliberate and often repeated administrations to the eye, and consequently they are designed to provide a pH, tonicity, and buffer capacity compatible with physiological limits. Under these conditions there is no reason to expect many ocular changes to occur after topical administration of these preparations, except for possible manifestations of sensitization or true toxicity of the drug. In fact, if one applies the Draize scoring system to eye preparations, the total mean score of 4 (which is the limit of detection of irritation) is rarely obtained, while the maximum possible Draize score is 110. This means that the scarcity, the mildness, and transientness of changes usually observed during the course of ocular irritation studies in laboratory animals with ophthalmic preparations do not raise the same kinds of ethical objections when testing chemicals and/or cosmetics. However, one of the major issues in any test conducted to evaluate hazards to human beings remains: How nearly does the test conducted actually predict a human response? We will try from a review of literature and from our own experience to address this critical issue. We will limit ourselves to ocular irritation per se, excluding sensitization and true ocular toxicity. We will also envision possible improvements and mention alternatives to the presently used test.

II. Tests Presently Used

Several reviews of tests currently used have been provided: Marzulli and Simon (1971) and later McDonald and Shadduck (1977) published overviews which summarize the state of the art of ocular irritation testing. The main advances are briefly summarized here.

Historically, the assessment of ocular changes after instillation of standard quantities of material into the eyes of laboratory animals, especially rabbits, relies on a subjective clinical observation of treated eyes and numerical grading of changes. These nonparametric data are added together to obtain a final score. The first scoring method widely used was proposed by Friedenwald *et al.* (1944) to study the acid–base tolerance of the rabbit cornea. Although the persistence of the induced changes was considered, this technique lacked sensitivity and was soon replaced by the Draize *et al.* (1944) scoring system, from which was derived the ocular test recommended by regulatory or governmental agencies (Draize, 1959; FDA, 1965; *Official Journal of the French Republic,* 1972). The Draize test consists of a time-dependent clinical follow-up of macroscopic changes induced in the cornea, the iris, and the palpebral conjunctiva since Draize *et al.* (1944) "decided to divide the overall effect into distinct elements." One eye only is treated; the other serves as control. In this test, special emphasis is given to the cornea as a transparent medium, but no attention is given to the other transparent media (aqueous humor, lens, and vitreous body). Macroscopic changes in the three above-mentioned ocular tissues are observed at different times and numerically graded according to a scoring system. The extent and/or seriousness of the tissue changes are considered at each observation point; numerical gradings are transformed by a formula into a final score evaluating the overall effects (the maximum score is 110). The Draize test published in 1944 usually included readings at 1, 24, and 48 hr after instillation and after 96 hr if "present residual injury" (Draize *et al.*, 1944). In later publications, readings included a 72-hr survey and were extended to hour 168 (Draize, 1959; cited in Kay and Calandra, 1962). These scores mainly allowed comparison of compounds. In 1965 the FDA proposed to use the test qualitatively to assess whether or not a compound was an ocular irritant, and this determination depended on the number of rabbits exhibiting a so-called positive reaction.

However, the subjectivity in grading ocular changes leads to variations in appraisals and scoring ocular reactions, and thus difficulties were encountered in the interpretation of obtained data. Reflecting the need for methodological analysis of the final scores, interpretative methods were proposed. Hoppe *et al.* (1950) recommended several daily appraisals of ocular reactions. Kay and Calandra (1962) proposed a three-step classification: the first two steps gave a temporary, provisional classification resulting from the mean values, and the third step determined the terminal classification of the test compound "considering the overall consistency of the data" (Idson, 1968) and balanced the temporary classification according to the distribution of individual scores. These techniques provided good results for compounds moderately to severely irritant—namely, industrial compounds—but lack sensitivity for very slight to slight graded irritant preparations (i.e., cosmetics and ocular preparations).

Different types of methodological improvements were made to assess more effectively subtle changes due to "weak" irritants and were especially applied for testing cosmetics and ocular preparations. They were intended to reduce the subjectivity of clinical macroscopic observations, and they usually generated more reliable data. They consisted of improvements of *in vivo* examination of ocular tissues, also applied to other transparent media of the eye; objective measurements included assessment of *in vivo* vascular permeability and postmortem examinations of ocular structures with increasing refinement of microscopic techniques. The main contributory improvements are here briefly summarized:

1. Detailed clinical study of onset (Hoppe *et al.*, 1950), persistence of lesions (up to day 14 of study; Scharpf *et al.*, 1972), recovery, and sequelae (Weltman *et al.*, 1965; Duprat and Gradiski, 1973).
2. Improvement of eye survey: naked eye observations replaced by use of an ophthalmoscope and/or slit lamp in rabbits (Weltman *et al.*, 1965; Baldwin *et al.*, 1973; McDonald *et al.*, 1973), also applied to other species (Buehler and Newman, 1964; Gershbein and McDonald, 1977). This equipment provides more detailed observations of the cornea and the iris, and also allows deeper investigation (aqueous humor, lens, vitreous body, retina, and optic disk).
3. Recording of additional objective parameters: at the time of eye survey, corneal thickness can be measured with an adequate device and provides a good index of stromal hydration (Burton, 1972; McDonald *et al.*, 1973); intraocular pressure can be recorded at that time directly by means of a tonometer (Ballantyne *et al.*, 1976), or after *in vivo* cannulation (Paterson and Pfister, 1974; Conquet *et al.*, 1977); corneal anesthesia can also be assessed. (The *in vivo* study of aqueous humor formation and outflow by fluorographic techniques is apparently restricted to more fundamental pharmacological studies.)
4. Systematic use of standardized clinical observations alone or in combination with elementary tests immediately after instillation; observation of bulbar conjunctival reddening (prominence of limbic vessels), measurement of frequency and duration of blinking, measurement of lacrimation (and not eyelid overflow) with blotting paper, or by length of wet fur.
5. Dynamic approach of minimal irritation by assessing increased capillary permeability after *in vivo* injection of a vital dye (e.g., Evans blue); this technique requires careful ophthalmological survey of palpebral and bulbar conjunctiva, cornea, and aqueous humor, and sequential determinations of dye concentrations in ocular tissues (Laillier *et al.*, 1975; Conquet *et al.*, 1977).
6. Study of the effect of lavage once (Draize, 1959) or at various times after instillation (Davies *et al.*, 1976), however, does not constitute a routine part of ocular testing, except for some cosmetics (shampoos, etc.).
7. Microscopic investigations: exfoliative cytology during the course of the study (Walberg, 1983), or postmortem examinations; microscopic evaluation of eyes (and adnexa), as proposed by Weltman *et al.*

(1965) to ascertain fully and record structural changes. This latter type of examination is now part of the toxicological screen for submission before release of the compounds to the public.

8. Use of refined morphological techniques *in vivo* (specular microscopy) or at termination (electron microscopy); since transverse sections are usually evaluated by light microscopy, scanning electron microscopy (SEM) providing three-dimentional images is recommended and has been developed. SEM can also be used *in vivo* for conjunctival and corneal cytological studies, but such a use of SEM has not been extensively reported (the utility of SEM will be covered in a later section). Specular microscopy is more often used for human clinical studies.

III. Are Tests Used Presently Predictive?

The only means to answer such a question accurately would be to conduct studies in human beings that are similar in every aspect to those performed in animals; of course, this is never done, particularly when preparations tested in laboratory animals induce side effects that outweigh the expected therapeutic benefit, because in this case, such preparations are not developed further. As a consequence, one finds on the market only products that satisfactorily pass the experimental stage, which really limits the question to "Are preparations found satisfactory in laboratory animals also found acceptable by millions of patients?" If one considers on one hand the millions of patients who daily use ophthalmic preparations and, on the other hand, the very low incidence of reported unpredictable ocular side effects, the answer is yes. In addition, to the best of our knowledge, no product has been withdrawn because of side effects which could not have been detected in animals with appropriate tests available at the time of drug development.

However, some side effects which do not preclude the continuation of a preparation's utilization are sometimes detected only after wide use by the public. Then, the answer to the question is probably better phrased as "yes, but." Let us take as an example the glaucoma market in the United States. Today, this market represents an average of 15 million prescriptions a year, and the number of reported ocular side effects clearly attributable to the use of antiglaucoma preparations, and which were not found during the course of preclinical and clinical investigations, is extremely low and in the range of parts per million. Speaking of antiglaucoma preparations, the development of timolol maleate in our laboratories has been for us the first opportunity, and we believe probably the first time in the pharmaceutical industry, to conduct very long-term ocular irritation studies with an ophthalmic preparation: 1 year in rabbits, 2 years in dogs. Several years after commercialization of this product, it is interesting to review the results of the preclinical evaluation and compare them with the ocular side effects detected during the course of clinical investigations prior to launching the product, and with those reported in the literature after millions of prescriptions written for human beings.

A. Review of Preclinical Ocular Safety Studies

1. *Preclinical Rabbit Study*

In the rabbit, timolol maleate ophthalmic solutions at 0.5 and 1.5% concentrations were administered to groups of 12 males and 12 females for a period of up to 12 months. Control rabbits were treated with the vehicle or physiological saline. Drug preparations and vehicle contained benzalkonium chloride (BAK) as a preservative at a 0.01% concentration. Four times a day, 0.1 ml of the preparation was instilled in the left eye of rabbits. The right eye served as an untreated control. At the end of the treatment period, animals were sacrificed under general anesthesia and postmortem examinations were done on eyes and adnexa. Ocular reactions based on Draize's scoring system were recorded daily, immediately before and after each instillation. Biomicroscopic ophthalmological examinations were performed before testing and before dosing in weeks 5, 9, 14, 21, 29, and 52 by Lionel Rubin, a veterinarian and consultant ophthalmologist.

The principal ocular reactions seen following administration of all preparations were mild transient conjunctival congestion which varied from animal to animal during each week of the study, but with a slightly higher incidence and intensity in the 1.5% timolol maleate-treated group than in other groups. There was no difference between vehicle and the 0.5% timolol maleate-treated group. The lower scores, however, were always observed in the saline group, as reflected in Fig. 1. Ophthalmic examinations did not reveal any change attributable to timolol maleate treatment. However, corneal roughening (Table I) was observed in treated eyes from all groups, but with a lower incidence in the saline group, which could tentatively be correlated to the presence of a preservative in these preparations. This will be discussed later.

Local anesthetic activity was also evaluated on the rabbit cornea.

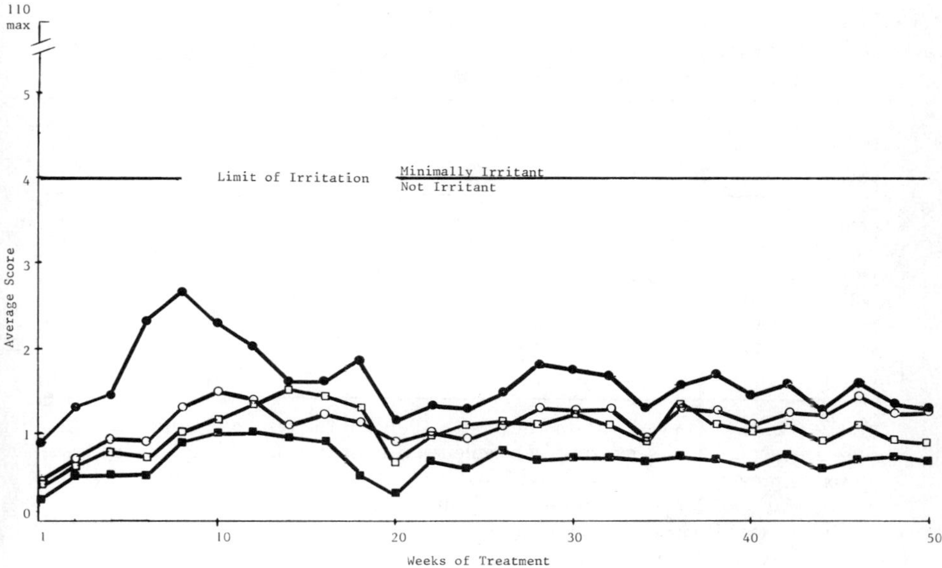

FIG. 1. Timolol maleate ophthalmic solution: 12-month ocular irritation study in rabbits. Average weekly scores, Draize scoring method. ●, 1.5% timolol maleate; ○, 0.5% timolol maleate; □, vehicle; ■, saline.

TABLE I

RESULTS OF A 12-MONTH OCULAR IRRITATION STUDY OF TIMOLOL MALEATE OPHTHALMIC SOLUTION IN RABBITS[a]

Treatment groups	Weeks of examination						Total number of animals involved
	5	9	14	27	39	52	
1.5% Timolol maleate	2	1	1	2	1	2	5 (3 females, 2 males)
0.5% Timolol maleate	0	2	1	2	1	4	6 females
Vehicle	1	0	3	0	0	4	5 (4 females, 1 male)
Saline	1	0	0	0	0	0	1 male

[a]Numbers represent numbers of treated eyes showing corneal roughening upon opthalmic examination. Note that one untreated eye from a control animal also showed this change.

TABLE II

LOCAL ANESTHETIC ACTIVITY ON THE RABBIT EYE: NUMBER OF TOPICAL STIMULI NEEDED TO INDUCE BLINKING REFLEX[a]

Compound[b]	Time (min)						
	0	2	5	8	10	20	30
Control	1	1	1	1	1	1	1
Saline	1	1	1	1	1	1	1
Oxybuprocaine, sale weight (0.4%)	1	> 200[c]	> 200	> 200	> 200	> 200	> 200
Timolol, base weight (1.2%)	1	3	2	1	1	1	1
Propranolol, base weight (1.3%)	1	24	29	41	38	4	1
Atenolol, salt weight (1.0%)	1	1	1	1	1	1	1
Pindolol, salt weight (1.0%)	1	2	5	14	10	5	9

[a]At $t = 0$ min, both eyes were instilled with 100 μl of the test compounds or saline. Results are means of three separate experiments. A nylon thread manipulated by hand was used to provide topical stimulation.

[b]Concentration given as percentage in parentheses.

[c]The count was stopped after 200 contacts.

Blinking was elicited by touching the cornea with tip of a nylon filament of 1 cm length (Cochet esthesiometer). Normally, the reflex took place after one stimulation, but, in the anesthetized cornea, repetitive stimuli were required. The effects of timolol maleate, propranolol hydrochloride, atenolol hydrochloride, pindolol tartrate, and, as a reference agent, oxybuprocaine hydrochloride, were studies after ocular application of doses effective in lowering intraocular pressure. The corneal anesthetic action of oxybuprocaine (0.4%) was clearly evident (Table II). In contrast, no evident local anesthetic effect followed instillation of saline, timolol, or atenolol. Propranolol induced a moderate corneal anesthesia which lasted for 10 min after topical administration. Pindolol exhibited a slight local anesthetic effect 5–30 min after its instillation. The results suggest that timolol maleate lacks corneal local anesthetic activity.

2. *Preclinical Dog Study*

In the dog, chronic studies constructed similarly to the rabbit studies were conducted over a 2-year period on four groups of 10 animals which received approximately 30 μl of the preparation three times a day. Slight transient hyperemia of conjunctivae occurred after instillation of all preparations. During the first month of the studies, frequency of hyperemia was about 100, 34, 14, and 4% for the 1.5%,

0.5% timolol maleate, vehicle, and saline groups, respectively. In the 0.5% timolol maleate group, incidence gradually increased up to 65% until the third month, when it remained stable. The duration of the hyperemia was usually less than 10 min in vehicle and saline groups, and 15–30 min in both timolol maleate groups. Blinking of the eye was also observed in most dogs from the 1.5% timolol maleate group, and in about 60% of the 0.5% timolol maleate group, and only occasionally with the vehicle and saline groups. These results clearly indicate that animals reacted mildly to the daily instillations of timolol maleate. However, as shown in Fig. 2, the Draize score obtained in the timolol maleate groups remained well under the limit of irritation. Ophthalmological examination failed to reveal any changes attributable to timolol maleate.

B. Clinical Situation

1. *Clinical Studies Conducted for New Drug Applications*

During these studies, timolol maleate ophthalmic solution, in a recommended twice-daily dose, with concentrations of 0.25–0 5%, was associated with few undesirable local side effects. The most common

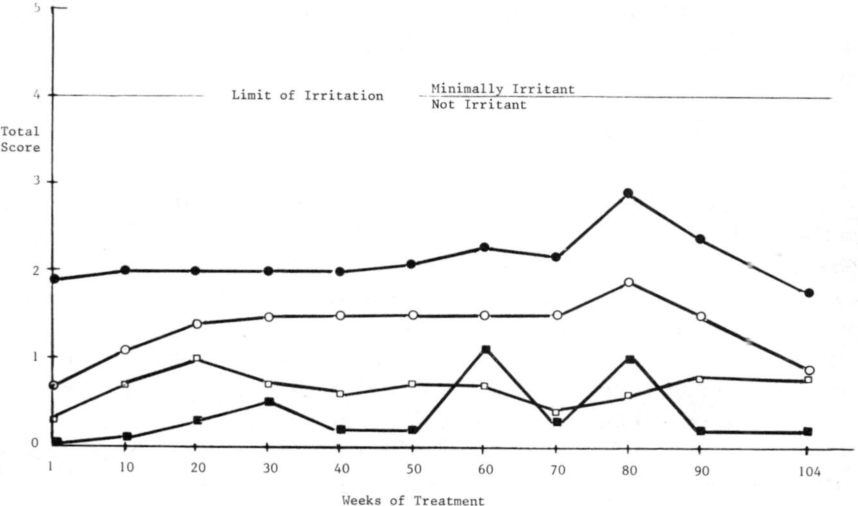

Fig. 2. Timolol maleate ophthalmic solution: 2-year ocular irritation study in dogs. Average weekly scores, Draize scoring method. Symbols as in Fig. 1.

local reactions for patients receiving timolol solution were transient ocular burning (9%) and blurred vision (7%). However, according to Katz (1978), blurred vision usually resulted from the elimination of the increased accommodation associated with prior myotic therapy, and thus cannot be considered as a side effect per se. None of these reactions was severe enough to cause patients to drop out of the study. Burning occurred less frequently in patients receiving 0.1–0.5% timolol maleate than with higher concentrations. Rare punctate keratitis occurred only in the early pharmacodynamic studies in which very frequent measurements of intraocular pressure were done using local anesthetic agents. These changes occurred in both treated and untreated eyes, indicating that the cause could not be attributed to timolol maleate ophthalmic solution. Such changes were not seen during the usual clinical routine therapeutic studies, when frequent or multiple daily pressure measurements were not often made. The Shirmer's test for tear production was done in several studies. The use of timolol maleate ophthalmic solution, for periods up to 1 year, was not associated with decreased tear formation.

The changes described above are very similar to those found in animals. In addition, humans, like rabbits and dogs, did not evidence any pupillomotor effect following timolol maleate treatment. It is clear that with this compound at least, animals were very good predictors of what happened on a population of approximately 1000 glaucomatous patients, but this was before the commercialization of the product, and it is interesting now to see what happened after the launch of the product.

2. Ocular Adverse Effects of Timolol Maleate Reported after Commercialization

Van Buskirk (1980) analyzed the 547 cases reported to the U.S. National Registry between October 1978 and September 1979 encompassing ocular and systemic effects possibly related to timolol maleate topical treatment. A quarter of these changes were external ocular side effects, resembling qualitatively and quantitatively those observed during clinical trials, with two exceptions. Nineteen cases of possible allergic reactions were reported in the National Registry but were not verified. Such reactions were never evidenced during preclinical and clinical investigations. There were also 12 cases of lost corneal sensitivity; such reactions were not reported during clinical investigation. These apparent discrepancies can be explained simply on the basis of the difference of scale.

Katz (1982) reviewed the adverse results reported by the Drug Experience and Epidemiology Department of Merck Sharp & Dohme Research Laboratories (MSDRL) for the first 3 years since timolol maleate was introduced in the United States (see Table III). During this period of time, it has been estimated that 700,000 patients representing more than 10 million prescriptions have been treated with this preparation.

Again, it is important to underline the very low incidence of external ocular side effects observed with this product when compared with the number of prescriptions, and again, the incidence as well as the nature of the changes observed correlate well with the preclinical and clinical findings.

Ocular irritation testing is an important step in the safety assessment of ophthalmic preparations. Despite anatomical dissimilarities, animal models are reliable and predictable, and significant technical improvements were made in the past decades. New morphological techniques might provide other significant advances in ocular irritation testing.

TABLE III

OCULAR EVENTS REPORTED: U.S. MARKET EXPERIENCE

Type of event	Number of events			
	1 Year[a]		3 Years[b]	
	No.	%	No.	%
Ocular irritation	72	43	198	51
Visual refraction	46	27	96	25
Corneal complications[c]	18	11	44	11
Other[d]	33	20	52	13
Total	169	100	390	100

[a]Reported to MSDRL between October 1, 1978 and September 30, 1979, estimate of 300,000 patients treated.

[b]Reported between October 1, 1978 and September 30, 1981, estimate of 700,000 patients treated.

[c]Edema, punctate keratopathy, keratitic precipitates, corneal ulcer, ground glass appearance.

[d]Abnormalities of conjunctiva, lens, uveal tract, pupil motility, retina, lids and adnexa.

IV. Can We Improve the Predictivity of the Tests?

From the timolol maleate preclinical and clinical data, sensitive and predictive animal models are available. Elegant morphological techniques (scanning electron microscopy and specular microscopy) have been introduced in ophthalmological research over the past decade. They are now routinely used for safety evaluation of ophthalmic drugs under development. From the literature and our own experience with preservatives, the usefulness of these new techniques is presented.

A. Scanning Electron Microscopy

In most countries, regulations require multidose ocular preparations to be marketed when suitable preservatives are incorporated in the formulation. The local effects of preservatives were extensively studied *in vivo* and *in vitro,* and scanning electron microscopy (SEM) had revealed preservative-induced morphological changes on the corneal surface, usually affecting the first epithelial cell layer, which is very important for exchanges between cornea and lacrimal film. These results are summarized, discussed, and put into perspective for the clinical human situation. Comparative effects of various vehicles and preservatives (BAK, thiomerosal, chlorhexidine, etc.), alone and/or in ophthalmic preparations, were largely studied on rabbit corneas. The local corneal effects were investigated by several authors, specifically with SEM (Gasset *et al.,* 1974; Gasset and Ishii, 1975; Tonjum, 1975; Pfister and Burstein, 1976; Burstein and Klyce, 1977; Green *et al.,* 1980; Dormans and Van Logten, 1982; Kilp and Brewitt, 1984), and cytotoxic changes were described with each preservative, but at different concentrations. The same sequence of epithelial cytotoxic alterations were seen: (1) partial and then total loss of surface microvilli and plicae, (2) membrane changes and loss of contact between contiguous cells, (3) wrinkling of dying cells, and (4) exfoliation (this process starts by single-cell peeling and extends to desquamation of groups of cells). The exfoliation usually affects the first superficial cell layer, exposing the underlying unaffected second epithelial cell layer (microvilli are visible), but at higher concentrations (10-fold or above the concentration used in ophthalmic preparations) the alteration may further affect the second cell layer or deeper.

This sequence, however, varies in time and intensity with each compound, but most published data agree with this time sequence of cellular events. For most authors BAK is the most potentially damaging in rabbits, and therefore was chosen as a positive control. These *in vivo* observations were also found during *in vitro* studies in rabbits (see Burstein review, 1980a) and in rats (Crouch *et al.*, 1985). These findings were confirmed in human cornea, *in vivo* (Gasset, 1977) and *in vitro* (Crouch *et al.*, 1985). And changes seen with the usual concentration of ocular preparations (BAK, 0.01%) might explain the preservative-induced increased permeability in human and rabbit corneas (Burstein, 1984).

However, results of all these studies require careful analysis and discussion before making a final statement and extrapolation to humans. One can discuss the relevance of experimental conditions to the human clinical situation, particularly the test species and number of animals in study, the concentrations used, the route of exposure, the frequency of instillations, the duration of exposure, and the total duration of the *in vivo* studies. In some experiments, the concentration of preservative studied (i.e., 0.05% BAK, Dormans and Van Logten, 1982) was far above the one normally used in ophthalmic formulations. And for this latter concentration, direct extrapolation of rabbit data to human clinical situation must consider the rabbit's physiological characteristics: it seldom blinks, does not lacrimate much, and has a nictitating membrane, a device for close contact and acting as a reservoir (Buehler and Newman, 1964). But Burstein (1980b), determining a cytotoxic threshold for BAK in two species—cats and rabbits—showed a no-effect level of 0.001% (this was reported or confirmed by some of the previously mentioned authors, while for others the no-effect level was 0.004%) in both species, which reacted similarly to the same preservative concentration.

Experimentally, rabbits, cats, rats, and monkeys react similarly to BAK under the same conditions. If we consider the time of exposure in most studies, including the large comparative study of Pfister and Burstein (1976), corneal changes were followed after acute, generally single, exposure. But of prospective interest was Dormans and Van Logten's observation (1982): after 2 and 8 hr of BAK at concentrations in therapeutic ophthalmic preparations (0.01%), "the corneas had the same appearance as after 30 minutes," which confirmed a previous observation of Pfister and Burstein (1976), who had observed similar damaging effects after 30 and 60 min (BAK, 0.05%). Our personal results (Figs. 3 and 4), obtained in albino rabbits with various concentrations of BAK (ranging from 0.05 to 0.0001%, 50 μl, three times a day, for 1 or 15 consecutive days, one eye treated and the contralateral eye serving as a control), confirmed the cytotoxic effects but clearly indicated that they did not progress with time (Conquet and Duprat,

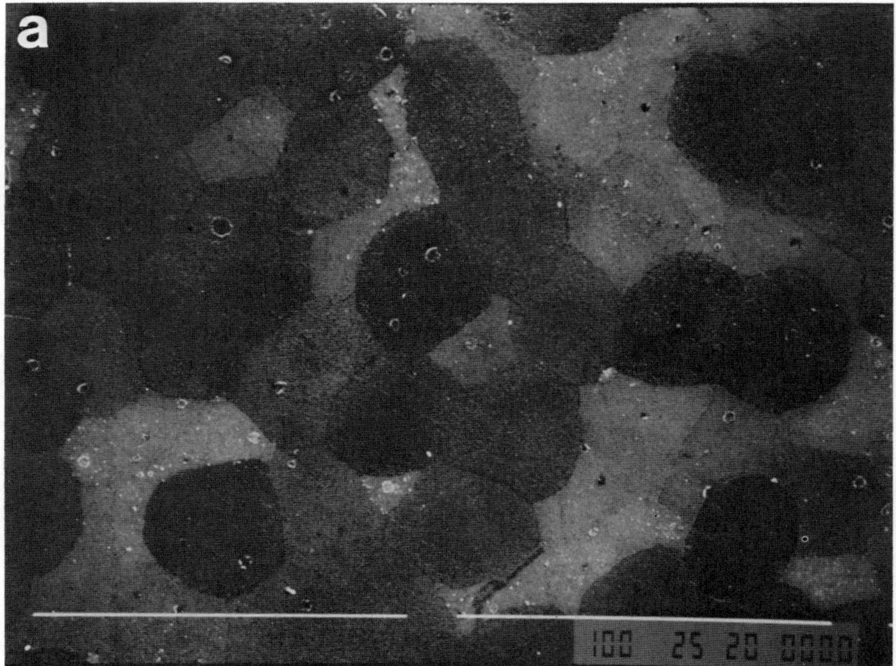

FIG. 3. Scanning electron micrographs (×500) of rabbit corneas; single-day study. (a) Control; (b) BAK 0.01% (50 μl, three times daily), no change; (c) BAK 0.05% (50 μl, three times daily), death of first epithelial cell layer and exfoliation.

unpublished data). These observations indicated that these epithelial alterations did not progress deeper and possibly underwent some recovery, since under light microscopy, Pfister and Burstein (1976) observed a thicker anterior epithelium that might be interpreted as undergoing reactive hyperplasia.

Considering the type of exposure of the test compounds in these previous studies, one can question the relevance of these data to the human clinical situation with daily use, and sometimes multiple daily instillations. The 0.001% BAK concentration experimentally determined *in vivo* as not damaging for the corneal epithelium is 10 times lower than the usual one of ophthalmic preparations. We know from worldwide use that 0.01% BAK has a great tolerance in humans, and that from guinea pig study, BAK has no sensitizing potential (Conquet *et al.*, 1984). This supports the SNIP's recommendation (1983) for multidose ophthalmic preparations of BAK concentrations between 0.005

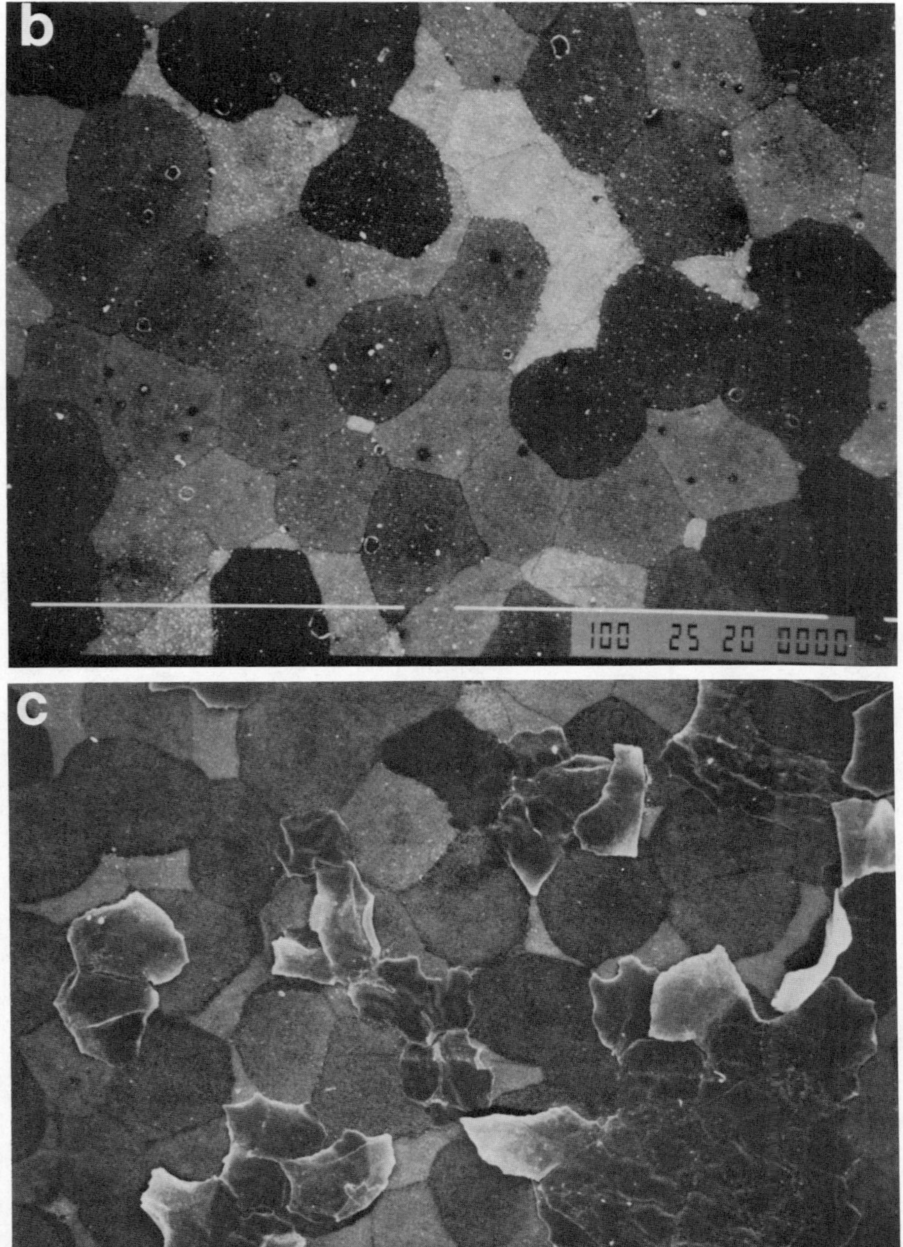
b
100 25 20 0000
c
100 25 20 0000

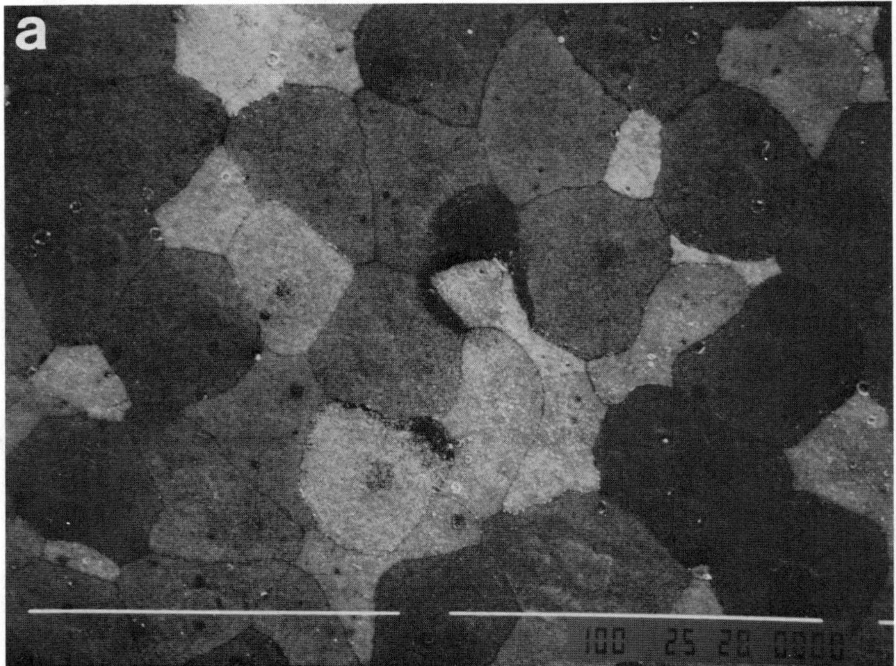

FIG. 4. Scanning electron micrographs (×500) of rabbit corneas; 15 consecutive days study. (a) Control; (b) BAK 0.01% (50 μl, three times daily), no change; (c) BAK 0.05% (50 μl, three times daily), death of first epithelial cell layer and exfoliation.

and 0.02%. Of interest was Burstein's description (1980a) of minimal spontaneous corneal individual surface changes, cell wrinkling, and minimal cellular exfoliation, which probably represents the normal turnover of epithelial cells in rabbits and that we found also equally or very slightly greater depending on the animal. In our study with a large number of control eyes, various degrees and frequencies of spontaneous single-cell peeling or multiple-cell desquamation were occasionally encountered, and this cell turnover might have been underevaluated (Conquet and Duprat, unpublished data). Moreover, Kilp and Brewitt (1984) reported minimal epithelial cell changes due to phosphate buffer solution application (30 min, 100 μl on the cornea). Thus, we can further speculate on an additive interfering effect of cell turnover with the test solution, since approximately every 4 days an increase in epithelial desquamation is known to occur in rabbits (Kikkawa, 1972).

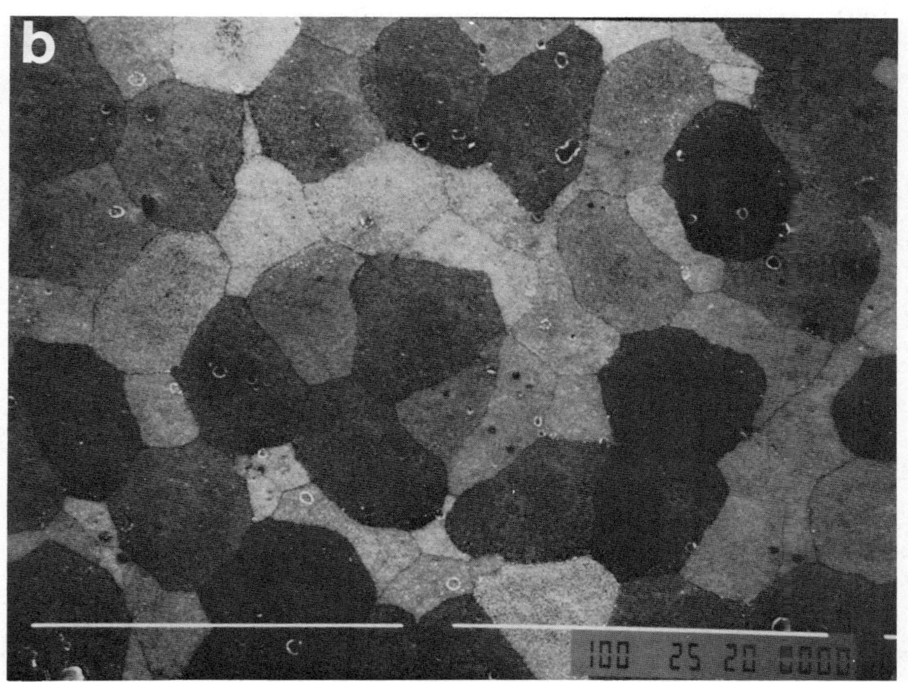
b
100 25 20

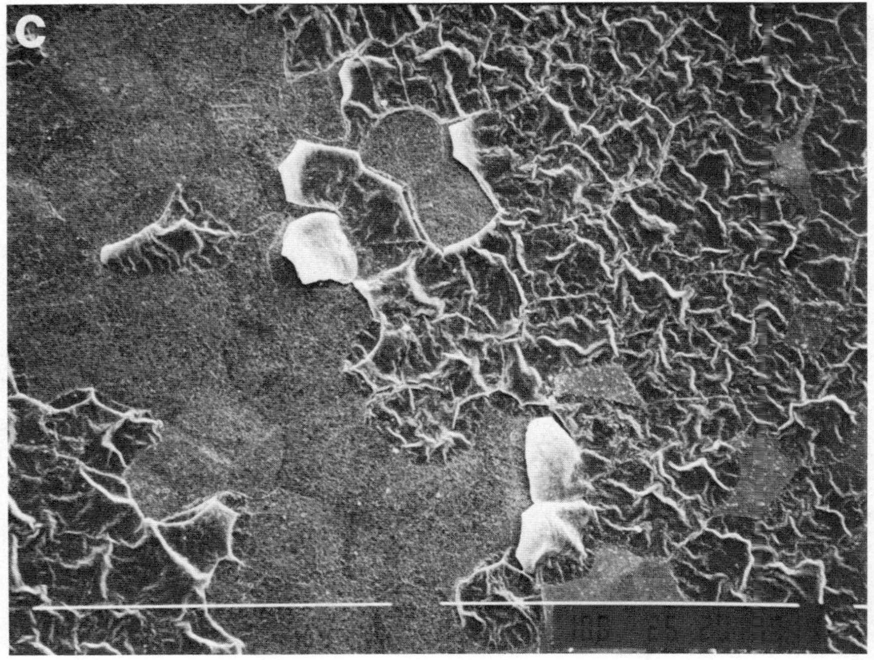
c

As a matter of fact, we can probably relate these findings with our own preclinical findings in the timolol maleate-treated rabbit in which all preparations containing BAK induced in a 1-year study a higher incidence of corneal changes when compared to the saline-treated group, and might explain the corneal roughening (Table I) seen in the preclinical rabbit study with timolol maleate in vehicle containing BAK (0.01%). Confirmation was given by Arthur *et al.* (1983), who studied the ultrastructural (SEM and TEM) effects of 1-month topical timolol on rabbit corneas, and by an *in vitro* study (Takkashi, 1983). He showed that commercial preparations of timolol maleate had in his experimental design a CDT_{50} much shorter than timolol maleate at the same concentration but without preservative. This seems to indicate that the effect observed is attributable to the preservative used. However, the change was so minimal that it was not taken into account in the interpretation, and also there were no changes of note in the dog study. There are very few other published results describing corneal surface changes in laboratory animals after drug instillation.

Minimal corneal changes were reported by Maudgal *et al.* (1981) with few commercial drugs (three drugs, with BAK 0.01% as preservative, instilled five times daily in the rabbit eye for 4 consecutive days). Alteration of the first epithelial cell layer was reported by Araki and Ogata (1980) with 1% bupranolol for 8 months in rabbits: exfoliation of cells was present at 3 months and at 8 months, and have had a limited progression. Because integrity and viability are important endothelial cell features for cornea transparency, the effects were also studied when preservatives were applied into the eye. On external application to the corneas, there were no endothelial changes (Conquet and Duprat, unpublished data). But important and sometimes irreversible endothelial changes have been caused by irrigation or perfusions with solutions containing these preservatives (Britton *et al.*, 1976; Levine *et al.*, 1979; Green *et al.*, 1980; Collin and Grabsch, 1982a,b). However, this did not reproduce physiological conditions and represented abnormal or accidental use (preparation not intended for surgical use).

Generally, the endothelial morphology can be followed *in vivo* during animal experiments or human disease. This feasibility probably explains why there is a limited number of SEM observations of this structure during tolerance studies. It is, however, noteworthy that SEM was frequently used in the fundamental study of endothelium repair and confirmed that the primate appeared to provide a better model than the rabbit cornea (Van Horn and Hyndiuk, 1975). Among new morphological approaches for ocular tolerance, SEM with high magnification capability allows evaluation of large areas and observation of minute cell surface details.

This provides a three-dimensional image of conjunctival and corneal surfaces. Normally, they are covered by microvilli (or microplicae), and cell borders and hole-like structures in the cornea, and various types of orifices (mucous glands, goblet cells, tear ducts in the conjunctiva). The SEM observation of the external ocular surface appears thus very sensitive and could be applied to *in vivo* and *in vitro* studies. Criteria for suitable tolerance—such as loss of microvilli, microplicae, increased spontaneous cellular desquamation above physiological threshold—must be set up, and more extensive studies of in-depth and surface damages should be routinely evaluated. But to be extrapolated to the clinical human situation, results must be obtained in relevant studies and, in other cases, the use of data should be restricted to comparison between several test compounds. We have to remember Burstein's philosophy (1980a): "Once extensive clinical experience is obtained in human without major deleterious effect, there is justifiable reluctance to rely further on animal experiments." However, this must not preclude further studies for improvements. Impression technique appears also to provide a rapid and simple *in vivo* technique to collect the greatest number of ocular cells (and inflammatory cells when present) to follow by sequential SEM observations of tissue response to topical application. Moreover, if SEM provides meaningful observations concerning the tolerance of topical application sites, it appears very useful to observe the trabecular meshwork, a very important structure in the aqueous humor outflow system. We recommend a more systematic use of SEM in ocular tolerance studies *in vivo* and in experiments with organ or cell cultures.

B. Specular Microscopy

Specular microscopy has been widely used in humans to study (1) the normal population of endothelial cells—morphology, density, and variation with age (Yee *et al.,* 1985) after repeated instillations of drugs (Alanko and Airaksinen, 1983); (2) repair capacity (Kaufman and Katz, 1977); (3) disease-associated changes; and (4) changes resulting from accidental trauma or surgery (keratoplasty, artificial eye lens implantation). Specular microscopy makes it easy to relocate abnormal features precisely and therefore facilitates long-term observations (as emphasized by Sherrard and Buckley, 1981; Lohman *et al.,* 1981) and allows study of the onset, time course, and reversibility of endothelial changes because the observed structures are "still alive." There is, however, little evidence in the literature of the routine use of a specular microscope in animal tolerance studies. This is probably because of difficulties in use. It lacks optical resolution (although an improvement was the development of wide-field equipment); the stability of images is limited and experimental in-depth studies require quantitative image analysis, a rather cumbersome method. Specular microscopy is still progressing and has been used in both applied and fundamental animal ophthamological research: (1) in applied research as a necessary tool to compare storage methods before corneal grafts (Laflamme, 1977; Campbell *et al.*, 1978) and to elucidate changes occurring during corneal storage (Sherrard, 1978), and as a complementary approach to assess the relevance of the animal model to human diseases (e.g., glaucoma: Ytteborg and Dolhman, 1965; Svedberg, 1975; Melamed *et al.*, 1980); (2) in fundamental research to study healing processes and mechanisms taking place in rabbit and cat endothelium (Olson, 1979). Regarding the potential *in vivo* use of specular microscopy, its use will probably increase in the future. Its use has recently been proposed to measure lens fibers *in vivo* (Bron and Lambert, 1984), which will certainly contribute to this growth.

In summary, both SEM and specular microscopy are very refined techniques in ophthalmic research to determine the adverse effects of compounds on the surface of the conjunctiva and the corneal epithelium and endothelium (Basu, 1983) and later to study the repair mechanisms (Gordon, 1983). They allow a better definition of general cell appearance and cell borders by means of three-dimensional images. In the near future they will probably be more often used in ocular tolerance tests, either during the course or at termination of the study. But since they are very sensitive, they should be limited to specific investigations and not used on a routine basis.

V. Can We Develop Alternative Methods to the Use of Animals?

Intensive efforts are currently being made throughout the world to develop alternative methods to *in vivo* eye irritation studies. A detailed and referenced review of all published data is not possible in this overview of ocular irritation tests, but research studies in this field should be briefly mentioned. Tests under investigation include morphological and cytotoxic techniques with cell cultures from different origins, use of multilayered membranes (e.g., egg chorioallantoic membrane) which represent a more elaborated barrier, use of corneal explants or eyes freshly removed, and use of isolated organs. Results of alternative methods show that they usually appear too sensitive: in corneal epithelium culture (rabbit wound closure model), BAK is cytotoxic at 0.001%, and the recommended concentration should be 0.0001% (Jumblatt *et al.*, 1985). Some of these techniques and/or results look promising, but no model mimics the *in vivo* situation and there is presently no consensus concerning one or a few of them. There is a great need for a reliable, simple, and inexpensive screening test, but investigations and search for correlations between *in vivo* and *in vitro* results have to continue. However, the exact purpose of *in vitro* toxicology and alternative methods must be clearly determined (Rowan and Goldberg, 1985). They must correspond to one of the four interfaces between *in vitro* and *in vivo* testing described by Nardone and Bradlaw (1983): "screening tests, mechanistic studies, personnel monitoring and considerations for risk assessment."

VI. Conclusions

The review of rabbit and dog preclinical data with timolol maleate ophthalmic preparation showed that these two models were good predictors of human response. This was confirmed by the pre- and post-marketing survey of patients undergoing antiglaucoma treatment, during which no major adverse effects were detected. The same correlation between animal observations and human clinical response has been seen with indocid ophthalmic preparation. The predictive value of animal models in ocular irritation is certain, documented, and validated.

We can use more sensitive techniques of examination and new methodologies for better evaluation of side effects of eye preparations, but prior to that, we must establish good correlation with clinical findings. It should be detrimental to the progress of therapeutics to eliminate potentially interesting compounds because of changes observed with inadequate, sometimes overly sensitive tests or methodologies.

Acknowledgements

We are grateful to Dr. Sylvain Molon-Noblot for the scanning electron-microscopic study and Ms. Blanche Robert for preparing the manuscript.

References

Alanko, H. I., and Airaksinen, P. J. (1983). *Am. J. Ophthalmol.* **96,** 615–621.

Anonymous (1964). Federal Food, Drug and Cosmetic Act. *Natl. Acad. Sci., Natl. Res. Council* No. 1138.

Anonymous (1971). Ministerial decree. *Off. J. Rep. Fr.* **April 21,** 3862–3864.
Araki, M., and Ogata, T. (1980). *Nippon Ganka Gakkai Zasshi* **84,** 1376–1384.
Arthur, B. W., Hay, G. J., Wasan, S. M., and Willis, W. E. (1983). *Arch. Ophthalmol.* **101,** 1607–1610.
Baldwin, H. A., MacDonald, T. O., and Beasley, C. H. (1973). *J. Soc. Cosmet. Chem.* **24,** 181.
Ballantyne, B., Gazzar, M. F., and Swanston, D. W. (1976). *Toxicology* **6,** 173–187.
Basu, P. K. (1983). *Indian J. Ophthalmol.* **31,** 476–485.
Britton, B., Hervey, R., and Kasten, K. (1976). *Ophthal. Surg.* **7,** 46–55.
Bron, A. J., and Lambert, S. (1984). *Ophthalm. Res.* **16,** 209.
Buehler, E. V., and Newmann, E. A. (1964). *Toxicol. Appl. Pharmacol.* **6,** 701–710.
Burstein, N. L. (1980a). *Surv. Ophthalmol.* **25,** 19–30.
Burstein, N. L. (1980b). *Invest. Ophthalmol. Vis. Sci.* **19,** 308–313.
Burstein, N. L. (1984). *Invest. Ophthalmol. Vis. Sci.* **25,** 1453–1457.
Burstein, N. L., and Klyce, St. D. (1977). *Invest. Ophthalmol. Vis. Sci.* **16,** 899–911.
Burton, A. B. G. (1972). *Food Cosmet. Toxicol.* **10,** 209–217.
Campbell, R. C., Bourne, W. M., and Campbell, R. J. (1978). *Arch. Ophthalmol.* **96,** 2108–2110.
Collin, H. B., and Grabsch, B. E. (1982a). *Acta Ophthalmol.* **60,** 93–105.
Collin, H. B., and Grabsch, B. E. (1982b). *Am. J. Optom. Physiol. Opt.* **59,** 215–222.
Conquet, Ph., Durand, G., Laillier, J., and Plazonnet, B. (1977). *Toxicol. Appl. Pharmacol.* **39,** 129–139.
Conquet, Ph., Duprat, P., and Plazonnet, B. (1984). *Poster Int. Congr. Eye Res., 6th, Alicante, Spain, Oct. 1–7.*
Crouch, R., Dennis, P., Neville, R., and Sens, D. (1985). *ARVO Abstr. Suppl. Invest. Ophthalmol. Vis. Sci.* **26,** 175.
Davies, R. E., Kynoch, S. R., and Ligett, M. P. (1976). *J. Soc. Cosmet. Chem.* **27,** 301–306.
Dormans, J. A., and Van Logten, M. J. (1982). *Toxicol. Appl. Pharmacol.* **62,** 251–261.
Draize, J. H. (1959). *Assoc. Food Drug Off. U.S.A.* 49–52 (Editorial Committee, Baltimore).
Draize, J. H., Woodard, G., and Calvery, H. O. (1944). *J. Pharmacol. Exp. Ther.* **82,** 377–390.
Duprat, P., and Gradiski, D. (1973). *Arch. Mal. Prof.* **13,** 265–269.
FDA (Food and Drug Administration) (1965). Proposal for qualitative use of Draize test. Washington, D.C.
Friedenwald, J. S., Hughes, W. F., Jr., and Hermann, H. (1944). *Arch Ophthalmol.* **31,** 279–283.
Gasset, A. R. (1977). *Am. J. Ophthalmol.* **84,** 169–171.
Gasset, A. R., and Ishii, Y. (1975). *Can. J. Ophthalmol.* **10,** 98–100.
Gasset, A. R., Ishii, Y., Kaufman, H. E., and Miller, T. L. (1974). *Am. J. Ophthalmol.* **78,** 98–105.
Gershbein, L. L., and McDonald, J. E. (1977). *Food Cosmet. Toxicol.* **15,** 131–134.
Gordon, S. R. (1983). *Eur. J. Cell Biol.* **31,** 26–33.
Green, K., Livinstone, V., Bowman, K., and Hull, D. S. (1980). *Arch. Ophthalmol.* **98,** 1273–1278.
Hoppe, J. O., Alexander, E. B., and Miller, L. C. (1950). *J. Am. Pharm. Assoc. Sci. Ed.* **39,** 147–151.
Idson, B. (1968). *J. Pharm. Sci.* **57,** 1–11.
Jumblatt, M. M., McLaughlin, N. J., and Neufeld, A. H. (1985). *ARVO Abstr.* p. 175.
Katz, I. M. (1978). *Proc. Int. Symp. Glaucoma, Int. Congr. Ophthalmol., 23rd, Kyoto, May 12.*

Katz, I. M. (1982). *Ophthalmol. Times* **7,** 1–26.
Kaufman, H. E., and Katz, J. I. (1977). *Invest. Ophthalmol. Vis. Sci.* **16,** 265–268.
Kay, J. H., and Calandra, J. C. (1962). *J. Soc. Cosmet. Chem.* **13,** 281–290.
Kikkawa, Y. (1972). *Exp. Eye Res.* **14,** 13–14.
Kilp, H., and Brewitt, H. (1984). *Chibret Int. J. Ophthalmol.* **1,** 4–20.
Laflamme, M. Y. (1977). *Can. J. Ophthalmol.* **12,** 128–132.
Laillier, J., Plazonnet, B., and Le Douarec, J. C. (1975). *Excerpta Med. Int. Congr. Ser.* No. 376, 336–350.
Levine, J. B., Binder, P. S., and Wickman, M. G. (1979). *Ann. Ophthalmol.* **11,** 1517–1528.
Lohman, L. E., Gullapalli, N. R., and Aquavella, J. A. (1981). *Am. J. Ophthalmol.* **92,** 43–48.
McDonald, T. O., Baldwin, H. A., and Beasley, C. H. (1973). *J. Soc. Cosmet. Chem.* **24,** 162–180.
McDonald, T. O., and Shadduck, J. A. (1977). *In* "Advances in Modern Toxicology" (F. N. Marzulli and H. I. Maibach, eds.), Vol. 4, Chap. 4, p. 139. Hemisphere, Washington, D.C.; Wiley, New York.
Marzulli, F. N., and Simon, M. E. (1971). *Am. J. Optom.* **48,** 61–79.
Maudgal, P. C., Cornelis, H., and Missoten, L. (1981). *Albrecht von Graefes Arch. Klin. Ophthalmol.* **216,** 191–203.
Melamed, S., Ben-Sira, I., and Ben-Shaul, Y. (1980). *Br. J. Ophthalmol.* **64,** 164–169.
Merck Sharp & Dohme Research Laboratories, Rahway, N.J. (1978). Timolol Ophthalmic Solution: Summary of Information.
Nardone, R. M., and Bradlaw, J. A. (1983). *J. Toxicol. Cutaneous Ocul. Toxicol.* **2,** 81–98.
Olsen, T. (1979). *Acta Ophthalmol.* **57,** 1014–1019.
Paterson, C. A., and Pfister, R. R. (1974). *Arch. Ophthalmol.* **91,** 211–218.
Pfister, R. R., and Burstein, N. (1976). *Invest. Ophthalmol. Vis. Sci.* **15,** 246–259.
Rowan, A. N., and Goldberg, A. M. (1985). *Annu. Rev. Pharmacol. Toxicol.* **25,** 225–247.
Scharpf, L. G., Hill, I. D., and Kelly, R. E. (1972). *Food Cosmet. Toxicol.* **10,** 829–837.
Sherrard, E. S. (1978). *Invest. Ophthalmol. Vis. Sci.* **17,** 322–326.
Sherrard, E. S., and Buckley, R. J. (1981). *Br. J. Ophthalmol.* **65,** 820–827
SNIP (Syndicat National de l'Industrie Pharmaceutique) (1983). Report by study group on "ophthalmic preparations." SNIP, 88, rue de la Faisanderie, 75782 Paris Cédex, France.
Svedbergh, B. (1975). *Acta Ophthalmol.* **53,** 839–855.
Takahashi, N. (1983). *Graefe's Arch. Clin. Exp. Ophthalmol.* **220,** 264–267
Tonjum, A. M. (1975). *Acta Ophthalmol.* **53,** 356–366.
Van Buskirk, E. M. (1980). *Ophthalmology* **87,** 447–450.
Van Horn, D. L., and Hyndiuk, R. A. (1975). *Exp. Eye Res.* **21,** 113–114.
Walberg, J. (1983). *Toxicol. Lett.* **18,** 49–55.
Weltman, A. S., Sparber, S. B., and Jurtshuk, T. (1965). *Toxicol. Appl. Pharmacol.* **7,** 308–319.
Yee, R. W., Matsuda, M., Schultz, R. O., and Edelhauser, H. F. (1985). *Curr. Eye Res.* **4,** 671–678.
Ytteborg, J., and Dolhman, C. (1965). *Arch. Ophthalmol.* **74,** 375–381.

Index

G

H

I

U

V

W